Communication Skills for Effective Dementia Care

Communication Skills for Effective Dementia Care

A Practical Guide to Communication and Interaction Training (CAIT)

Written and Edited by
Ian Andrew James and Laura Gibbons

Jessica Kingsley *Publishers*
London and Philadelphia

First published in 2019
by Jessica Kingsley Publishers
73 Collier Street
London N1 9BE, UK
and
400 Market Street, Suite 400
Philadelphia, PA 19106, USA

www.jkp.com

Library of Congress Cataloging in Publication Data
A CIP catalog record for this book is available from the Library of Congress

British Library Cataloguing in Publication Data
A CIP catalogue record for this book is available from the British Library

ISBN 978 1 78592 623 5
eISBN 978 1 78592 624 2

Printed and bound in Great Britain

How do you communicate effectively with people with dementia?

*People with dementia do not have 'special needs',
they have the same needs as the rest of us.*

*Owing to changes in their mental and physical abilities however, we
must be more creative in the ways we meet their needs. (James, 2018)*

Contents

Preface

Effective communication is critical for everyone and this book teaches the skills needed by healthcare staff in their day-to-day interactions with people with dementia (PWD) and their families. We illustrate the key aspects of communication that contribute to the development of a skilled and confident workforce, thus improving the effectiveness of the care provided.

Healthcare providers in the UK employ the largest workforce in Britain, one of the largest labour forces in the world. However, training gaps and a severe lack of funding for training and support by specialist teams is evident, particularly in dementia care. As clinicians who have worked with care homes for over 20 years, we have learned to appreciate the vital role good communication plays in maintaining the wellbeing of PWD. Over the years, we have collaborated in some of the major UK research programmes on the use of non-pharmacological treatments for behaviours that challenge (BtC), and recognise the importance of negotiation and de-escalating skills in reducing stress and distress in both PWD and their carers. Further, we are aware that staff deal with such behaviours on an hourly basis and thus they have acquired a range of effective skills in dealing with problematic situations.

This book is in two parts:

Part I: The first six chapters describe the CAIT (Communication and Interaction Training) framework developed by the authors. We use the components of a wheel to structure CAIT's contents, from the hub to the rim. In successive chapters we describe more sophisticated ways of interacting, although always drawing upon the core communication skills described in the hub. Indeed, we recognise that if we get the core communication correct, more complex interventions will not be required.

Part II: Here we have three chapters written by invited authors who are experts in specific areas of communication related to dementia and provide practical insights in relation to their specialisms. In Chapter 7 Susannah Thwaites introduces us to the work of Teepa Snow and Snow's framework known as the Positive Approach to Care™, which is a guide to effective communication and training for care-givers. Luke Tanner outlines his ideas on the importance of appropriate touch in Chapter 8, with a specific focus on obtaining informal consent prior to engaging in personal care. He examines the various types of touch and their relevance in positive interactions (Tanner, 2017). Chapter 9, written by Maggie Ellis and Arlene Astell, provides a unique perspective on how to communicate with people in late stage dementia. Their approach is known as 'Adaptive Interaction' (Ellis and Astell, 2017). In the final chapter, Chapter 10, we provide an overview of the recent national guidelines and research studies that have led to the upsurge in interest in care-giver communication skills over the last few years.

This is the third in a series of texts on dementia (see James, 2011; James and Jackman, 2017). The earlier books focused entirely on BtC and were written for an academic readership, containing psychological theories with detailed referencing. While complementary, the current book has a more practical orientation and tries to keep the referencing to the essential articles and book chapters. This book is intended to be also accessible for those, such as family members, who may not have any formal training in dementia care. The latter issue is important because the majority of PWD live in the community (two-thirds of PWD in the UK) and the communication of family members, or its absence, is crucial in terms of people's wellbeing.

Throughout this book we will discuss the importance of identifying and meeting people's needs. In dementia care, the idea that problems are usually a product of people's needs not being met is well established (i.e. unmet needs, Algase *et al.*, 1996; Cohen-Mansfield, 2000). It is relevant to note, however, that in our clinical work we have found a poor and inconsistent understanding of the nature of needs amongst carers. If we do not agree what needs are, how can we attempt to meet them? Hence in this book we provide a finite list of needs that we believe are fundamental to PWD and everyone else. We then suggest, through information we provide, that we adopt styles of communication designed to meet the needs in our list and thereby reduce problems and enhance wellbeing.

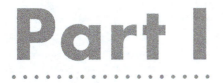

Part I

Chapter One

Introduction to CAIT

One of the key aims of CAIT is to reduce levels of stress and distress in PWD. Such agitation frequently occurs because of poor communication and often results in the prescribing of tranquilising and sedating medications (James and Jackman, 2017). Our clinical work shows that the strategies we recommend in this book have a double-impact: (i) they reduce the likely occurrence of behaviours that challenge (BtC); and (ii) they help de-escalate situations in which the person with dementia has become distressed or agitated.

KEY CONCEPTS OF CAIT
Best practice in communication
Best practice indicators (Health Education England, 2018) state that staff need to be able to establish rapport, undertake active and empathic listening, and be non-judgemental. Our training endeavours to promote awareness of the values and actions that services need to employ to reduce potential barriers to effective communication and develop the competencies required to deliver good care (James and Hope, 2013).

Strength-based relationship (SBR) approach
The contents of this book are based on observations of the good practices we have witnessed by staff. Hence, it is our intention to highlight these skills and build on them, rather than introduce a set of brand new approaches. For this reason we have called CAIT a 'strength-based relationship' (SBR) approach. We intend to build on staff's existing strengths without being patronising.

The goals of the SBR method may appear straightforward; however, there are two barriers to its use: (i) staff are usually unaware of the complexity of the skills they employ in difficult situations, and when asked about the skills they possess they have great difficulties articulating them (Carper, 1978); and (ii) once competencies are highlighted, however, staff may say 'we know all of this already', and can proceed to dismiss the value of our training.

Based on our experience, we feel it is important that staff become aware of the skills they possess, so they can take credit for good work and improve in any areas that they are struggling with (e.g. a carer may be really good at undertaking intimate care activities with men with mild dementia, but struggles with those with severe dementias, who have language difficulties).

Further, we understand that the staff are already undertaking many of the approaches we are going to be teaching, but our intentions are to improve and fine-tune existing competencies. We also want staff to articulate what they regard as being best practice across a range of situations, such as meal times and assisting someone to the toilet, and achieve consistency in approaches across the workforce. As with any workforce, there is a range of abilities in members of a team and our role is to ensure everyone is working to a good consistent standard.

Scenarios

This book has been written with the following typical scenarios in mind:

- Communicating well with people in everyday situations; treating PWD with respect and dignity during the normal course of daily living. Reducing the likelihood of stress and distress in PWD through the way we speak and interact.

- Using good communication skills to persuade PWD to undertake essential activities to maintain their wellbeing, including going to the bathroom, changing soiled clothing, getting out of bed and taking medication, particularly in circumstances they do not want to carry out these tasks.

- Communicating with people who become agitated and distressed temporarily and using good de-escalation strategies to deal with their temporary difficulties.

- Working with people who are repeatedly engaging in BtC; undertaking comprehensive assessments and interventions; developing formulations and effective care plans.

CAIT structure

CAIT is built on basic communication principles and includes advanced evidence-based treatment strategies for the management of BtC. CAIT's structure is represented visually in the form of a wheel, with the hubs, spokes, and rim (Figure 1.1, James, 2015).

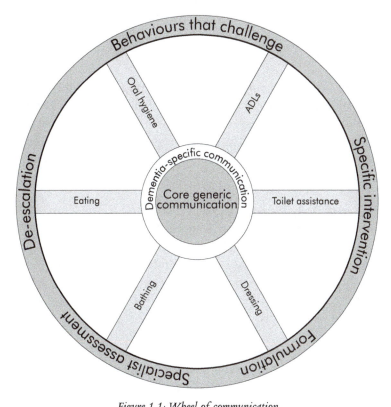

Figure 1.1: Wheel of communication

Aspects of the 'Wheel of communication' are discussed in the next five chapters, which are reviewed below.

Understanding People's Needs (Chapter 2)

This chapter outlines the importance of understanding people's needs and presents details regarding what we actually mean by a need. We also examine two of the main conceptual themes that reoccur throughout the book: the first is Cognitive Behaviour Therapy (CBT) and the other is being able to Reduce the emotion, Assess the need and Meet the need (RAM).

General Communication: Inner Hub (Chapter 3)

One could perhaps assume that healthcare staff working with PWD, especially in long-term care facilities, receive basic communication training; however this is not the case in many settings. Our training in this chapter is built around the central skill of good, basic, respectful communication. Such skills are similar to those taught to retail staff and law enforcement officers around customer care. We believe that ensuring staff are using empathic, considerate communication will reduce the need for some of the more advanced strategies.

Dementia Specific Communication: Outer Hub (Chapter 4)

We examine the adaptations required to communicate with PWD. The nature of dementia is discussed, together with the skills needed in day-to-day interactions, such as: body-language, appropriate pacing, use of personal space, types of questions to use/avoid, and persuasion and negotiation skills.

Activities of Daily Living (ADL) and
Levels of Functioning: Spokes (Chapter 5)

Staff are often supporting people to undertake personal hygiene activities. Owing to the intimate nature and potential invasiveness surrounding ADLs, these activities often trigger BtC. To minimise distress and agitation, we highlight the hands-on carer skills required to manage and navigate daily living in a sensitive, dignified and empathic manner.

Formulation-led Approaches: Rim (Chapter 6)

Here we teach the advanced skills used to manage problematic behaviours that arise from time to time. This may involve the use of specialist management and assessment techniques. Materials from the Newcastle Behaviour Support Team are used within this part of the teaching, including assessment methods, formulations, charts and interventions.

The CAIT programme is currently being delivered with the assistance of Tyne and Wear Care Alliance across the North East of England. In our current training programme all of the care homes in the Sunderland locality (N=60) are receiving CAIT in phases over a period of three years, supported with extensive supervision. All of the material presented in this book has been employed during our teaching and supervision with our Sunderland colleagues.

SUMMARY

We have introduced the components of CAIT and discussed its philosophy. Further we have suggested that if staff get the core communication skills right at the beginning of CAIT, the more sophisticated strategies may not be required. This is because the PWD will be being spoken to in ways that make them feel respected, cared for, listened to, and in control of themselves and their environment. The latter features are some of the basic human needs required for people to feel content. In contrast, however, when such needs are not met, people will often become stressed and distressed.

This notion of people not having their basic needs met is believed to be common in dementia care (Algase, *et al.*, 1996; Cohen-Mansfield, 2000); it is often referred to as the 'unmet needs' phenomenon. Cohen-Mansfield has linked the problem to agitation and distress in PWD, and others have identified it as a common trigger for BtC (Kitwood, 1997). Over the course of this book we will be looking at how best to meet people's needs through effective communication and positive interactions.

Chapter Two
....

Understanding People's Needs

This chapter outlines the importance of understanding people's needs and presents details regarding what we mean by a need. We examine two of the main conceptual themes that reoccur throughout the book: the first is the Cognitive Behaviour Therapy (CBT) approach which helps carers to understand the thoughts and feelings of PWD, thereby allowing carers to identify people's needs; and the second is being able to Reduce the emotion, Assess the need and Meet the need (RAM). RAM's three-step approach is complementary to CBT and is used for de-escalating situations that have the potential to become confrontational. RAM guides carers to respond calmly and intelligently rather emotionally and provocatively.

MEETING THE NEEDS OF PEOPLE LIVING WITH DEMENTIA

Cohen-Mansfield (2000) states that many of the behaviours we label as problematic are expressions of unmet needs. Using this view, she says that whenever we witness a BtC, we should check: (i) is the behaviour a reaction at wanting to be free from pain or discomfort? (ii) is the person's behaviour an action to fulfil a desire or goal? (iii) is the behaviour reflecting frustration at not being allowed to fulfil a need? (see Figure 2.1).

Several researchers and clinicians have examined the nature of needs and devised useful classification systems (Glasser, 1990; Kitwood, 1997; Maslow, 1943). A very helpful explanation was given by Tom Kitwood, who talked a lot about promoting people's wellbeing by meeting their needs, and his tool known as Dementia Care Mapping assesses wellbeing in care settings. Kitwood believed that we could prevent distress, and the emergence of problematic behaviours, through creating physical and social environments that promote quality of life. He represented the key components of his positive psychology in terms of the petals of a flower (Figure 2.2).

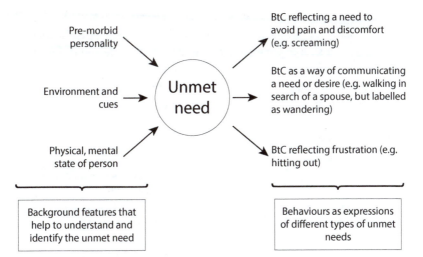

Figure 2.1: Cohen-Mansfield's notion of unmet needs

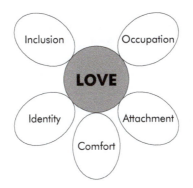

Figure 2.2: Kitwood's Flower of Needs

Another well-known model was developed by Maslow, who introduced us to the idea of a five-tier hierarchical model of needs, from basic food and shelter to self-fulfilment themes. Maslow (1943, 1954) stated that people are motivated to achieve certain needs and that some needs take precedence over others. Our most basic need is for physical survival and this will be the first thing that motivates our behaviour. Once that level is fulfilled the next levels become the foci: safety, belonging, esteem and self-actualisation. Whilst a helpful concept, the newer versions of Maslow's framework are complex and pay insufficient attention to an individual's wishes for other people's needs. Indeed, there seems to be no place for altruistic needs in the Maslow framework (i.e. putting other people's needs before our own).

In an attempt to keep things simple and relevant, and taking our lead from care staff, we produced a table of needs composed of eight themes (Table 2.1). This table amalgamates the previous models and describes themes that are common throughout the literature. The list is an expression of the eight underlying needs that are related directly to the occurrence of BtC when they are not satisfied (i.e. unmet needs).

Table 2.1: Classification of needs in dementia care

Fundamental needs	Expressions of someone whose needs are not being met (a wish, demand, request, statement)
Physical comfort and freedom from pain – air, food, shelter, sleep and freedom from pain.	Can you help; Will you give me something to eat or turn the temperature up?
Perception of safety – having a sense of security in terms of health and safety. Not wishing to feel fearful, vulnerable, nor having worries about health.	Go away; I'm afraid, I want to leave; Can I come along with you? I'm scared.
Positive touch – gaining pleasure from meaningful physical touch with another person.	Will you hold my hand? Let me give you a hug.
Love and belonging – the need for relationships, social connections, to give and receive affection and to feel part of a group. To have a sense of inclusion.	I want to spend more time with you; Please don't leave me; Do you still love me?
Esteem needs – feeling valued, treated with dignity and respect. To be recognised as competent, to be skilled, to be recognised for achievements and skill, to be listened to and have a sense of self-worth. Linked to sense of identity.	Don't you dare speak to me as if I am a child; Don't boss me around.
Control over environment and possessions (freedom) – the need to be free is the need for independence, autonomy, to have choices and to be able to take control of the direction of one's life.	Get out of my house; This is my chair; You can't come into my room; I want to go into the garden now.
Fun – the need to find pleasure, to play and to laugh.	I want to join in; I love going to parties; Shall we play a trick on him?
Occupation and exploration – the need to be active, to exercise curiosity, exploration. The need to have meaning and predictability in our lives.	I want to go to work; I want to see what is behind that door; Have you got something for me to do?

Case study: Unmet needs driving behaviour

Cathy was living with her husband, George, in their own home. George reported her increasing tendency to argue and occasionally hit him. Cathy had also started to try to run away, and on one occasion had climbed over the garden fence attempting to escape from George. She had also recently sworn at a taxi driver, who had been escorting her back to the house after Cathy became confused during a shopping trip. George had responded to these difficulties by trying to keep his wife in the house and taking over the running of the home.

From the use of assessment charts, we recorded increasing episodes of verbal aggression and arguments over household chores, self-care activities and finances. Cathy appeared to be particularly annoyed by being told what to do, where to go and what to wear by George. From his perspective, the only way he could cope with the situation was by trying to exercise tight control over the situation. Following a detailed review of the circumstances, we identified Cathy's unmet needs as:

- Lack of control over environment and possessions: Cathy, a proud, independent woman, wanted to feel she had some control over her life and environment.

- Threat to self-esteem needs and sense of powerlessness: She wanted her choices respected and acted upon.

- Lack of meaningful activity and occupation: Cathy did not perceive herself as having problems and wanted to continue to lead an interesting life and to contribute to the household duties.

The situation improved significantly when some of her needs were met by looking for ways of increasing her sense of control in her day-to-day activities and encouraging her to do household chores (no matter how poorly or slowly). Support was also provided for George, helping him to become more flexible and less controlling.

PWD's needs can be expressed both for the self and for others that they care for, including the desire to feel loved, have good self-esteem and have fun. They will become emotional, angry, depressed or low if these needs are not achieved for themselves or those they love and care for. This notion of the needs of others is crucial in dementia care and has not commonly been highlighted in previous frameworks that have described people's needs.

In the next section we look at two techniques for both identifying and also dealing with needs. The CBT framework examines the experience of people using a holistic perspective from which a need can be hypothesised based on people's appearances, speech and behaviour. The RAM framework is somewhat similar but also provides carers with guidance on how to deal with situations driven by needs that could potentially become confrontational.

THE CBT MODEL AND ITS RELEVANCE TO NEEDS

The CBT model represents people's experiences in terms of thoughts, feelings and behaviours (see Figure 2.3). Throughout this book we will regularly be checking out PWD's behaviours in relation to their feelings and style of thinking. Previously, PWD's cognitions were often ignored and seen as irrelevant owing to the disorientated and confused nature of their thinking. However, we believe that it is often the confusion and misinterpretations that result in problematic behaviours. Further we suggest that if we pay close attention to PWD's apparently 'non-sensical' language and appearance we will be better able to identify their needs and try to meet them as best we can.

Here is the script of someone with dementia, demonstrating his experiences in terms of the thoughts and emotions via the CBT cycle:

I woke up to at 5.30am to get out for the early shift down at the docks and the b*stards wouldn't open the door for me. They said they couldn't find the key. The liars, it makes me so angry. If I don't get to work I'll be in trouble with the foreman. I gave one of the women standing by the door a thump, but she still didn't let me out.

Figure 2.3 provides an example of the use of the CBT model, using the above scenario to examine the PWD's experiences and why this resulted in a BtC. Looked at in terms of needs, by examining the four features of the cycle we are better able to identify what unmet needs might be driving the behaviour.

We will now look at each of the features of the CBT cycle, illustrating why it is important to use the CBT features of behaviours, emotions, thoughts and physical sensations when learning to communicate better with people perceived to be challenging.

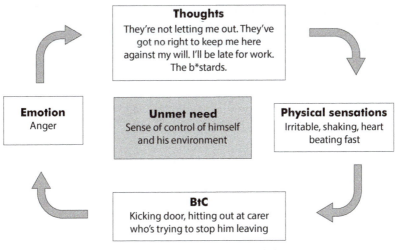

Figure 2.3: Going on the early shift

Behaviours

It is important not to over-pathologise BtC, and to be able to identify which behaviours require interventions. Table 2.2 lists behaviours taken from an audit of the work of the Newcastle Behaviour Support Team (James, 2010). As one can see, the actions listed are not unique to dementia. We daresay that these activities are common night-life phenomena of UK high streets on a weekend. Hence, we should not pathologise the actions of PWD and thereby rely only on a 'medical' model of treatment which is likely to involve medication. A meaningful investigation of why someone is acting in a way which could be seen as problematic would require gathering background information regarding the circumstances, including details about what was happening in the past and present, and environmental aspects.

It may be useful to see BtC as coping strategies used by the PWD to deal with their memory or physical difficulties. From such a perspective, we can reframe excessive walking as an attempt to deal with disorientation, or disrobing as a method for dealing with poor regulation of body temperature, and/or aggression as misperception of a threat.

Table 2.2: Table of behaviours

Aggressive forms of BtC	Non-aggressive forms of BtC
Hitting	Apathy
Kicking	Depression
Grabbing	Repetitive noise
Pushing	Repetitive questions
Nipping	Making strange noises
Scratching	Constant requests for help
Biting	Eating/drinking excessively
Spitting	Over-activity
Choking	Pacing
Hair pulling	General agitation
Tripping someone	Following others/trailing
Throwing objects	Inappropriate exposure of parts of body
Stick prodding	Masturbating in public areas
Stabbing	Urinating in inappropriate places
Swearing	Smearing
Screaming	Handling things inappropriately
Shouting	Dismantling objects
Physical sexual assault	Hoarding things
Verbal sexual advances	Hiding items
Acts of self-harm	Falling intentionally
	Eating inappropriate substances
	Non-compliance
	Misidentifying

The role of emotions in dementia care and BtC

One of CAIT's core concepts is recognising and responding to changes in emotional states. Ideally, healthcare staff will strive to maintain positive emotions in PWD, such as happiness, joy, pride and contentment, and reduce the negatives, including anxiety, anger, frustration or jealousy. This section discusses the relevance of emotions in dementia care and their relationship to good communication.

The three emotions most frequently associated with BtC are anxiety, anger and depression. Cognitive therapists such as Beck (1976) tell us that anxiety tends to happen in all of us when we think we cannot cope and see ourselves as being vulnerable. Anxiety is greatest when people see the environment as being chaotic and the future unpredictable. PWD are sometimes unable to say they are anxious; however, this emotion is very easy to identify from their facial expression. Anxiety is one of the six universal, pan-cultural emotions that we can recognise in people even if we do not speak their language. The other basic emotions we can recognise by facial expressions are happiness, surprise, sadness, anger and disgust.

Anger is an emotion that is easily identified. Beck (1976) tells us that anger tends to happen when people feel their rights are being infringed (i.e. they are being unjustly controlled). Therefore, as soon as you see someone getting angry, carers need to ask themselves what might be happening for the person to make her think that she is being taken advantage of. With this in mind, carers may then be able to think of ways to calm the person down.

Depression is associated with thoughts of worthlessness and hopelessness for the future. PWD may be unable to talk about their feelings, but if they look depressed, one needs to instil a sense of hope and do something to make life feel worthwhile. The best ways to do this is to help the person do things that they previously found enjoyable, perhaps using music, conversation or activities.

Thoughts

Thoughts have a major influence on how people feel and experience their world (James and Hope, 2013). We all have particular styles of thinking and our own likes, dislikes and worries, and we will see these reflected in how people behave. The thinking feature of the cycle is often the one most closely related to needs, as it is often an indication of how people are interpreting their current situation: *'Someone has stolen my purse'; 'Where are my children?'; 'I don't like it here, I want to go home.'*

In terms of dementia, people's behaviour may become inappropriate or unusual because of changes in their styles of thinking due to: (i) memory problems; (ii) confusion, misinterpretation or disorientation; and/or (iii) lack of insight. The combination of these features can be particularly problematic.

RAM (REDUCE THE EMOTION, ASSESS THE NEED, MEET THE NEED)

CAIT has an overriding framework known as RAM in which each letter represents a key element for delivering good care (see Figure 2.4). Whilst CAIT provides structure, the unifying thread that unites the features is RAM. The concept of needs, and the manner in which people's needs are met, is fundamental to RAM.

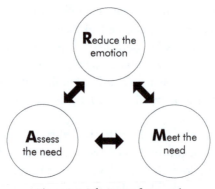

Figure 2.4: The RAM framework

If the person is initially upset because her needs are not getting met, the first step for a staff member is to calm her down (i.e. reduce the emotion); only then will she be receptive to working collaboratively towards a mutually positive outcome. This framework stresses the importance of identifying and meeting PWD's needs. For example, and as prompted by RAM, we encourage healthcare staff to form positive relationships, connect, listen and assess what people's needs are. Whilst all of these features may seem simple and straightforward, performing these interactions with PWD can often be complex. Although our primary goal is to help people get their needs met, sometimes we cannot meet them completely and we have to manoeuvre and meet them through indirect means, such as substituting the need, redirecting or creating a new need that will satisfy the PWD.

The amount of work required within each feature of RAM will differ depending upon the characteristics of the person and the nature of the BtC. At times more comprehensive assessments may be required, and on occasions this will constitute the use of a formulation. Formulations are person-centred descriptions of the person and her environment that are used to help understand the potential causes of the BtC. In terms of CAIT, more in-depth assessment and input are required in the later stages of the CAIT wheel (Chapter 6).

SUMMARY

In this chapter we have discussed the importance of meeting PWD's needs, and the association of unmet needs with problematic behaviour. The roles of CBT and RAM frameworks were discussed; CBT helps us to understand the nature of people's needs, and RAM provides practical ways of identifying and dealing with people's needs.

Chapter Three

General Communication: Inner Hub

This chapter is designed to introduce the key concepts and principles that underpin effective interpersonal interactions for all of us and not just for PWD. We use the term 'clients' because we are not necessarily always referring to PWD. We have drawn from numerous organisations in which good communication skills and training are an essential part of the employees' jobs. To this end, we discuss the training routinely given to both people working in high street stores (customer care skills) and law enforcement officers (Verbal Judo).

CUSTOMER CARE SKILLS

We can learn a lot from good customer care. General skills taught to shop assistants across the country are designed to ensure that customers have a good experience when shopping in retail stores. The staff are taught how to approach and speak to customers and deal with any problems or complaints.

The acronym CARES is used to summarise the five key features of good customer care skills that are employed in high street stores in the UK. Shop assistants are taught these techniques in their induction programmes at good quality retail shops. We believe that if these skills are appropriate to teach on the high street, they should be essential in care settings to ensure we too have satisfied service users and family members.

CARES

C – Making a Connection

Members of staff should use the clients' names often. They should inform the client who they are because this creates an immediate connection.

Interactions are often better when we are speaking to someone we know and feel we trust.

It is also important to employ effective body language. It is estimated that approximately 55 per cent of communication is body language, 38 per cent is the tone of voice and 7 per cent is the actual words spoken (Mehrabian, 1972, 1981). Adopt an open body stance, avoid standing immediately in front of the client, as this can be perceived as provocative, and try not to invade the client's personal space without his permission.

A – Active listening and Assessing the person's need

Staff can demonstrate they are listening through body language, for example, nodding, making good eye contact and by asking clarifying questions. Once we know what the person needs or wants, it is helpful to feed back one's understanding of the situation to show the client's difficulties are being taken seriously and there is an appreciation of the key concerns.

It is easy to misinterpret what someone wants or needs. For example, if a client says 'I need to go', you may incorrectly assume they want to leave the building, when really they want to go to the toilet. Clarify your understanding of the request, e.g. 'You say you "need to go", tell me about that?' Note how the client's own statement is repeated, and then more information is asked about the statement.

R – Reduce agitation and develop the Relationship

One of the first rules of negotiating is to reduce any anger or agitation to enable a calm conversation to take place. Once things are calm, the ability to form a good relationship with the client is crucial. In retail settings, staff are taught to engage quickly with their customers and to be friendly and respectable, thus forming a good relationship and partnership.

Within a healthcare setting, in order for a client to be able to disclose distress or to allow staff to give support with intimate tasks, there must be both trust and confidence in the carer. However, it is important that the relationship remains professional too, because staff have a code of conduct that must be adhered to.

E – Empathy

Empathy is the ability to make clients aware that their difficulties are being understood. It is important not only to understand what a client says, but also how he/she feels. The way we use empathy is also important; our empathy should not reinforce hopelessness or pessimism (*'Yeah, that is so bad I don't think I could cope with that either'*).

We have noticed, however, that good staff have the ability to use empathic skills to predict how someone may react or feel towards a given situation, and thereby manoeuvre the situation, preventing the person becoming distressed. Good staff also seem to be able to show understanding of difficulties, while offering solutions and optimism (*'I can see you're struggling with that, why don't we try doing it this way?'*).

S – Solve the problem by meeting the client's needs

When clients are asking for assistance, they have an issue or need they want resolving. Having assessed this, we should try to keep their frustration to a minimum. It is important that we give the client the impression that we have a solution to their difficulties, and we will also take time and care to resolve their issues.

The CARES framework is a simple and useful checklist. We believe that if the principles are applied most of the needs we identified in the Needs table (Table 2.1) would be fulfilled.

COMMUNICATION SKILLS FOR DEALING WITH CONFRONTATION

In this section we examine the communication skills required to deal with situations when confrontation has arisen. We introduce 'Verbal Judo', as used by police departments in the USA, and show how the RAM framework can be applied.

Verbal Judo

Verbal Judo, also called 'tactical language', highlights the requirement to control the emotional tone of any argument. George Thompson developed this form of communication for the police in the USA (Thompson and Jenkins, 2013). He warned against becoming emotionally over-involved in confrontations because we then become less rational; this is when the 'primitive brain' takes over, inhibiting our ability to be effective problem solvers (The Incredible Hulk vs Mr Spock).

Thompson's helpful tips include:

- Communicate calmly, even when others are upset and angry.

- Take control of the situation using calm, appropriately assertive language.

- Show respect; give reasons for your own behaviour rather than just saying 'NO'. For example, *'Please stop kicking the door for a moment, I want to see how I'm going to help with whatever's upsetting you.'*

Thompson says that arguing is likely to inflame the situation. Hence, initially it is helpful to try to calm the client and to demonstrate that you are able to understand someone's perspective rather than contradict it. The ability to project empathy is crucial to this de-escalation process. In Chapter 2, we discussed how people's emotional appearance (depression, anxiety, anger) can give major clues to their thinking styles. We encourage staff to use this information and their body language to tune into the client's perspective, and demonstrate that you have sympathy and understanding of their distress.

In Verbal Judo there are certain expressions we should avoid when dealing with agitated individuals, because such phrases have been shown to increase conflict (Table 3.1).

Table 3.1: Verbal Judo's unhelpful expressions

Unhelpful things to say to someone who is agitated	Helpful equivalents
Come here!	Hi Joan, would you mind coming over while I ask you a question?
What's your problem?	Can I help with something?
Because those are the rules	The reason I am asking you to do this is because of X and Y.
I'm not going to tell you again.	Would you mind listening carefully to this, because it's really important that we all understand what's happening.
What do you want me to do about it?	Tell me again about the problem, I will see if I can help.
Calm down.	I can see this is upsetting you.

(Adapted from DTM Security, 2015)

The concept of Verbal Judo shares features with the therapeutic approach known as Transactional Analysis (TA) (Berne, 1964). This is a well-known form of psychotherapy that tries to explain conflict between people by looking at how they speak to each other. Such analyses often reveal that individuals get upset when they feel someone is trying to either control or patronise them during the conversation. In TA terms this is referred to as a parent to child interaction. The preferred way of speaking in most situations is adult to adult, which displays mutual respect. The use of this approach is currently being applied to dementia care (James and Caiazza, 2018a).

De-escalation skills: The use of RAM

In Chapter 2 we introduced the RAM framework (Figure 2.4). In this section we show how RAM is helpful in confrontational situations, when the heightened emotional state makes people aggressive or defensive. The three features of the RAM are similar to the CARES and Verbal Judo frameworks discussed above.

When dealing with any form of agitation, it is important to attempt to calm the situation down. With training we can learn to *respond* to situations, rather than *react* to them, because reactions are often not well thought through and thus can make things worse. When we are responding well we are able to reduce the amount of energy in the interaction, permitting all parties to talk more rationally.

We must be able to keep our own emotions in check, even when provoked. This needs to be thoroughly rehearsed, for example through role playing of de-escalation scenarios (Thompson and Jenkins, 2013).

Reduce the emotion

At this stage there is a need to control the emotional tone of any argument. This involves:

- Connecting with the person, stating his name as well as your own. Connecting should be done in a genuine and empathic manner, creating the bond that will permit meaningful engagement.

- Sticking to the facts of the current situation. Do not either generalise (*'You always do this'; 'People like you can't help themselves'; 'It's typical of your family'*), or dig up the past (*'You did the same last time'; 'When we first met you would never have done that!'*). By going off-topic you provide the person with new ammunition to widen the dispute; the client can now argue about the past or the generalisations you have made.

- It is better to use statements that start with 'I' rather than 'You'. This prevents you being accused of mind reading by the other person, and makes you take responsibility for your own emotions and thoughts (for example, I think you dislike me vs You dislike me; I am feeling upset vs You are upsetting me; I feel stupid when I'm with you vs You make me feel stupid).

- Avoiding saying 'Calm down', as it tends to make people less calm.

- Avoiding starting a statement with negatives (e.g. *'You shouldn't have done that'; 'That is not allowed'*). If you say *'I understand'* you need to demonstrate that you are listening and trying to understand.

Arguing is likely to inflame the situation. Initially it is helpful to try to calm people and to demonstrate your ability to understand their perspective rather than contradict it. Being able to project empathy is crucial to the de-escalation process. Use people's statements and their body language to tune into their perspective, and demonstrate you have sympathy and understanding of their distress.

Assess the need

Clients are more likely to engage with you and stop pushing their view if you demonstrate you understand their perspective and have listened to their side of the story. However, as well as understanding their view, you need to convey your understanding in a helpful manner (aka tactical empathy). Helpful tips include:

- Listen and avoid pointing holes in their argument.

- Use powerful reinforcing statements, such as: *'Let me see if I understand what you've just said…'*

- Use empathic statements, which show that you are being attentive and trying to understand the concerns. It also gives the client opportunities to clarify his concerns: *'So I can see you're feeling X (upset, sad), is it because of Y (you've seen new bruises on your mother's arm)? Have I understood that correctly?'* In this case a family member can say, *'No, I'm feeling angry because another resident is wearing her new cardigan.'*

The latter types of statements are both empathic and help to identify the clients' needs – i.e. what they want to happen next. Some more useful empathic assessment phrases to help elicit what the client needs include: *'That's interesting…tell me more about that?'*; *'What makes you say that?'*; *'What makes you ask that?'*; *'What makes you want that?'*

These phrases must be said in a supportive, inquisitive manner and should not appear patronising or accusatory. These queries give you time to think about what to do next and give you a better assessment of the situation and the client's needs. Sometimes it may be necessary to help the client clarify what they want (aka 'Giving them ground to stand on'). For example, in the case of the family member who sees a fellow resident wearing her mother's cardigan, the immediate 'want' is related to the cardigan. However, the underlying need might be concerns that the staff are not treating her mother as an individual and not giving her due respect.

At the end of the needs assessment phase it is helpful to summarise the need and share this with the client, because this creates clarity and a platform for setting out a plan to meet the need.

Meet the need

When you have asked relevant questions, clients can now feel listened to and you can jointly start to think of ways of meeting their needs. Try to give them what they want or something approximate to this. This stage is often more difficult than it first appears and there may be some manoeuvring required. We are usually dealing with multiple needs – client's, staff's, manager's, organisation's, society's. The skill is to try to do justice to them all in an ethical and effective manner.

Before discussing needs in terms of PWD, it is worth highlighting that physical difficulties will influence the methods required to meet people's needs. For example, the authors (James and Hope, in preparation)[1] are currently interested in how relationships change when one is involved in a conversation in which you are seated and the other person is standing. This is a common event in dementia care settings, where the majority of residents spend over 80 per cent of their waking-time in a seated position, whether a wheelchair user or not. Early results show that the power imbalance sets up a whole series of dynamics that undermine the seated person's self-esteem and perception of control.

SUMMARY

If you are armed with the skills outlined above, you should be able to ensure members of the public feel respected and listened to even when complaining. The members of the trained workforce will give the impression that they are trying their best to resolve problems. We think, therefore, that if managers of retail stores and the police consider basic skills training is important, so should we!

In a study we conducted with care homes it was recognised amongst staff that interpersonal skills differed widely between them. Indeed, carers believed they could predict which of their colleagues were likely to make matters worse if they were ever involved in trying to resolve a confrontation (James *et al.*, in preparation).[2] Hence, we think that basic training in communication skills is both sensible and relevant for all carers to ensure effective, safe and consistent interactions with PWD.

---

1   Details can be obtained from the first author. CAV, Westgate Rd. Newcastle upon Tyne. NE4 6BE.

2   Details can be obtained from the first author. CAV, Westgate Rd. Newcastle upon Tyne. NE4 6BE.

Chapter Four

Dementia Specific Communication: Outer Hub

In this chapter we build on the communication skills outlined in Chapter 3 and discuss adaptations for people living with dementia. We highlight the features of dementia – the intellectual, sensory and physical changes associated with it – that make changes in verbal and non-verbal interactions necessary.

We also examine the skills required in day-to-day interactions and look at some of the reasons why we need to change the way we communicate with PWD when they are displaying agitated behaviours.

WHAT IS DEMENTIA?

The dementias are a group of diseases, such as Alzheimer's, vascular, dementia with Lewy body and frontotemporal dementia. They are characterised by an accelerated and progressive dying of brain cells, leading to mental, emotional and physical problems. The risk of being diagnosed with a dementia increases with age. Dementia is uncommon in people under the age of 60 but it can appear in people in their 40s or younger. Recent studies suggest that the actual disease process may begin in many people ten or more years before the first symptoms appear.

According to the Alzheimer's Society, there are 850,000 PWD in the UK, with numbers set to rise to over one million by 2025. This will soar to two million by 2051. This year 225,000 people will develop dementia – that is one every three minutes – and there are 40,000 people under 65 with dementia in the UK.

Knowing the different types of dementia and their presentations assists us to adapt and tailor our communication and interaction skills to the individual person. The features of each dementia are most evident in the early stages of the diseases; over time the types of dementias start to look like each other, owing to the cumulative impact of the deaths of so many brain cells.

There are also conditions called the pseudo-dementias, which present like dementia but are potentially reversible. They are caused by delirium, mental health problems, dehydration and malnutrition, severe constipation, and side-effects and interactions of drugs. Each of these conditions can cause confusion and disorientation and may lead onto distress and agitation in PWD. It is also important to highlight that often someone may be experiencing more that one of these features, leading to a complex negative cycle in which the problems become conflated. The initial step of all BtC treatment protocols should be the screening, usually by primary care services (e.g. general practitioners), for the above health conditions (James and Jackman, 2017).

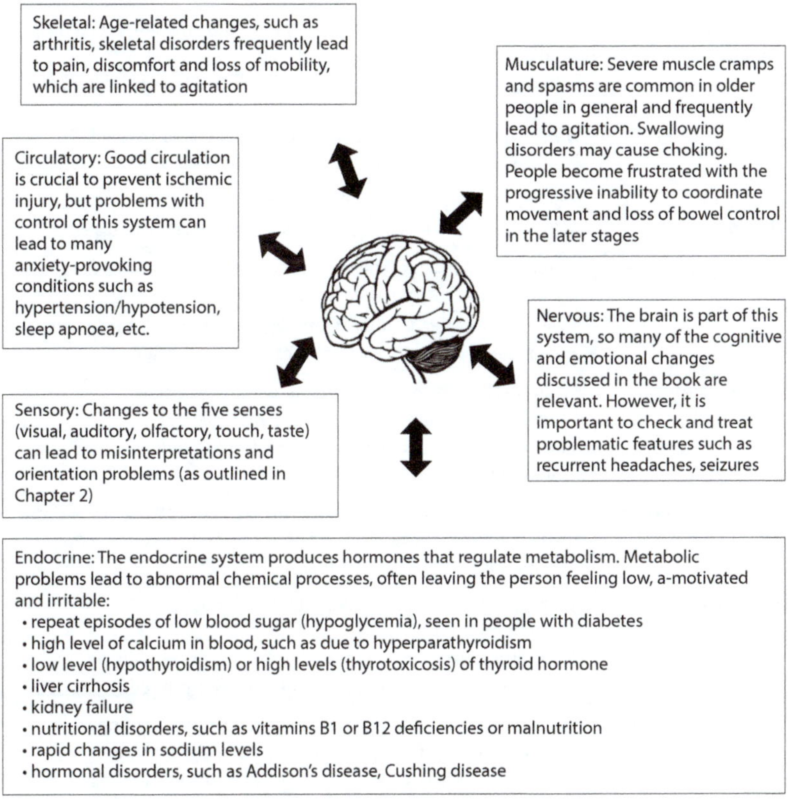

> Skeletal: Age-related changes, such as arthritis, skeletal disorders frequently lead to pain, discomfort and loss of mobility, which are linked to agitation

> Musculature: Severe muscle cramps and spasms are common in older people in general and frequently lead to agitation. Swallowing disorders may cause choking. People become frustrated with the progressive inability to coordinate movement and loss of bowel control in the later stages

> Circulatory: Good circulation is crucial to prevent ischemic injury, but problems with control of this system can lead to many anxiety-provoking conditions such as hypertension/hypotension, sleep apnoea, etc.

> Nervous: The brain is part of this system, so many of the cognitive and emotional changes discussed in the book are relevant. However, it is important to check and treat problematic features such as recurrent headaches, seizures

> Sensory: Changes to the five senses (visual, auditory, olfactory, touch, taste) can lead to misinterpretations and orientation problems (as outlined in Chapter 2)

> Endocrine: The endocrine system produces hormones that regulate metabolism. Metabolic problems lead to abnormal chemical processes, often leaving the person feeling low, a-motivated and irritable:
> • repeat episodes of low blood sugar (hypoglycemia), seen in people with diabetes
> • high level of calcium in blood, such as due to hyperparathyroidism
> • low level (hypothyroidism) or high levels (thyrotoxicosis) of thyroid hormone
> • liver cirrhosis
> • kidney failure
> • nutritional disorders, such as vitamins B1 or B12 deficiencies or malnutrition
> • rapid changes in sodium levels
> • hormonal disorders, such as Addison's disease, Cushing disease

Figure 4.1: Brain function and the gradual impact of disease processes

The brain coordinates many different functions of the body as shown in Figure 4.1, synchronising a vast network of bodily systems both unconsciously and consciously. Figure 4.1 presents some of the difficulties that can be experienced by the person when problems start to arise with the various functional areas. Some of the difficulties are age related, but losses are accelerated because of the premature dying of brain cells due to the dementias. As problems begin to develop, PWD struggle to do many things that they used to be able to do automatically, such as dressing or knowing when to go to the toilet.

As noted above, as more cells die the difficulties experienced by PWD will look very similar. A summary of the features that differentiate the common dementias is provided in Table 4.1. We need to be able to work with such changes when we are trying to communicate with PWD.

Table 4.1: Features of the common dementias

Areas of Change	How the changes are experienced by PWD
Memory changes	Better with older memories than newer ones – so often preferring to talk about the past. Reliving the past (person thinks she's still got young children, or is still at work). Worse with words and verbal memories compared to familiar activities and skills (muscle memory largely intact).
Language difficulties	Problems finding words, understanding things said. Better with sign-language or gestures than spoken language.
Hearing changes	Unable to understand sentences, particularly if long or spoken quickly, or said in a noisy environment. Increasingly unable to filter out background noise and focus on relevant speech, making comprehension very difficult.
Visual changes	Reduced vision, and gradual loss of peripheral vision. An inability to judge speed of things approaching. Loss of 3-D vision, leading to problems judging depth. Misinterpretation of visual information.
Olfactory changes	Food can taste or smell different bringing about change in appetite. Smells can become intense or overpowering. PWD often report smelling burning rubber or a fire.
Impulsiveness	Acting quickly without thinking things through. Taking more risks. Disinhibited, being rude (saying hurtful things, sexually inappropriate), talking loudly, being more self-centred.
Fine motor skills	Unable to manipulate fingers in small movements, leading to difficulties with self-care, eating and other daily activities. Unable to manipulate toes, leading to an odd gait, walking on ball of foot and difficulties manoeuvring (walking backwards).
Overactive fear response	Having a heightened 'fear' response. Constantly anxious and worried. Anxiety can sometimes lead to aggression/agitation.

Concentration/ attention	Difficulties focusing on things. Easily distracted, particularly in busy environment.
Insight	Poor insight, thinking everything is fine. Refusing help. Occasional insight to the fact they have dementia, leading to despair.
Slowed thinking	Difficulties working things out. Difficulties making decisions or understanding questions.

In a previous book in this series on dementia (James and Jackman, 2017, p.22) we discussed in detail the impact of these changes on PWD's functioning. In our 2017 text we highlighted how problems with people's vision, hearing, sense of smell, memory, speed of processing information or problem-solving have profound effects on the way PWD comprehend, relate to others and express themselves. Furthermore, whenever any of the problems outlined in Table 4.1 occur together, the person can really have difficulty undertaking tasks done easily in the past. This situation is made doubly difficult if the PWD no longer have insight that they are struggling to do things for themselves. In such circumstances, it is easy to see why we get BtC. Indeed, for this reason BtC are often quite predictable, as can be seen in the scenario outlined in Figure 4.2.

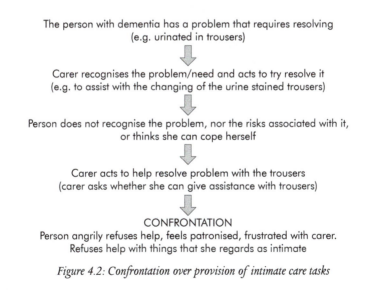

The person with dementia has a problem that requires resolving
(e.g. urinated in trousers)

Carer recognises the problem/need and acts to try resolve it
(e.g. to assist with the changing of the urine stained trousers)

Person does not recognise the problem, nor the risks associated with it,
or thinks she can cope herself

Carer acts to help resolve problem with the trousers
(carer asks whether she can give assistance with trousers)

CONFRONTATION
Person angrily refuses help, feels patronised, frustrated with carer.
Refuses help with things that she regards as intimate

Figure 4.2: Confrontation over provision of intimate care tasks

Poor insight can lead to other difficulties, particularly when the PWD is experiencing memory problems too. Indeed, the combination of these two features can lead to PWD behaving in unusual and frustrating ways, such as asking the same questions repeatedly and trying to carry out tasks they did in their pasts (i.e. time shifting – wanting to pick up their children from school or go to work). In order to understand such features, we first need to examine the nature of behaviour and how it relates to memory.

Behaviour (what we do and say) is determined by several features, including personality, context, environmental cues and our appraisal of the current situation. The appraisal will be based on our long-term memory (LTM), being in similar situations in the past, and short-term memory (STM), judgements about what has been happening during the last few minutes. By combining both we can determine whether we are OK or whether there are physical or emotional risks that we need to be concerned about. If things are judged to be risky, we can take actions (fight or flight responses).

We frequently choose to take decisive actions when we judge that our fundamental needs are not being met (i.e. we feel threatened, over controlled, excessively bored). In the case of PWD the same decision processes happen, but their STM is compromised and thus they are unable to recall what has just happened or what has just been said to them. PWD therefore tend to over-use information from LTM when making decisions about what to do next; they are frequently matching the current situation with similar scenarios from their past to help guide future actions. In that sense they are constantly using out-dated information to guide themselves in the 'here and now'.

The above features account for the two common phenomena of repetitive questioning and time shifting. Carers should be aware of these issues and their causes; such knowledge will help them deal with these two phenomena successfully, because these phenomena are often associated with BtC when handled badly.

In the next section we will discuss how to identify and approach people who are either repeating the same questions or re-living events from their past.

COMMUNICATING WITH PWD

In this section we discuss communication in general and also in relation to when someone is displaying agitated behaviours. Understanding language can be difficult even when our brain is functioning well. We recognise this sometimes when we visit parts of the country with distinctive accents. We find people difficult to understand because the locals are putting different stresses on parts of their words, speaking too fast, running words into each other, and using odd phrases and/or abbreviations. Now imagine what it is like to decipher speech when your brain is not working well, you are not hearing clearly, your thinking is slow and your STM is poor. It is for these reasons that PWD may be misunderstanding the majority of sentences spoken to them, although for the sake of saving face they may nod and pretend they comprehend.

In the initial stages of dementia we will see word finding difficulties, and problems with complex written and verbal sentences. People will use many words to make a point when only few words are needed. Later people will show naming deficits for the names of everyday objects (nouns), make errors in sentences and show decreased use of gestures. They will substitute words that sound alike, e.g. kippers for slippers. People with advanced Alzheimer's disease may lose the ability to initiate conversation. Echolalia – people repeating back to you what you have said – is possible.

We need to have an awareness of these deficits and learn to adapt our approach depending on a person's level of communication skills and thinking. Communication deficits can lead to frustration, self-isolation, reduced self-esteem and self-worth and BtC, and we need to remind ourselves of the key needs of PWD (Table 2.1) in order not to violate their needs during our interactions.

Case study: PWD isolating herself due to sensory problems

Maya was 79 and was diagnosed with Alzheimer's disease five years ago. During the first few years she remained the matriarchal figure in a close knit family. She had also continued to be the life and soul of any family gathering. However, six months ago there was a marked social change, whereby Maya started to sit at the edge of any family group and stopped joining in with conversations. At first this seemed confusing because she was very talkative when spoken to one-to-one. After a discussion with the specialist, it became evident that she had started to experience hearing difficulties. Indeed, although her ears were still functioning well, her ability to understand lots of voices at the same time had reduced.

She was also having difficulties tracking conversations from person to person as they told stories and jokes. Owing to reductions in her ability to process information quickly and efficiently, she became functionally deaf during family gatherings, unable to understand what was being said. As a result, she had begun to withdraw, which had a knock-on effect in terms of her sense of confidence and competence.

The following sections provide guidance on how to communicate with someone with dementia across a range of scenarios.

PREVENTATIVE STRATEGIES FOR MAINTAINING GENERAL WELLBEING
Approach

Approach slowly from the front and pause to make eye contact before entering the person's personal space. Once you have got the person's attention speak clearly and slowly. Use short sentences in a quiet environment that is not over-stimulating.

The slow approach is required because of the slowed thinking speed of the person. In Northern Europe and North America the boundary point for entering someone's personal space is approximately 4 feet; therefore pausing at this boundary prevents the person becoming overly anxious (Sorokowska *et al.*, 2017). Coming from the front is relevant owing to the difficulties of peripheral vision. Waiting to obtain eye contact ensures the person is prepared to interact with you. Teepa Snow refers to this method of approach as 'Connecting' (see Thwaites, Chapter 7).

The term 'brain blindness' is sometimes used to explain situations where the eyes continue to function, but the part of the brain responsible for visual processing (occipital lobe) has been damaged (Houston, 2015). The brain's capacity to interpret visual stimuli it receives from the eyes is decreased causing the following forms of visual impairments:

- narrowing of visual field, leading to reduced peripheral vision

- loss of depth and speed perception

- problems with pattern recognition

- double vision

- visual hallucinations.

We need to have an awareness of how these visual changes may affect a person's ability to interact with other people and her environment (Banham and Soares, 2017).

The use of short simple sentences means the person's comprehension skills are not over-taxed, and the quiet environment aids with attentional and concentration difficulties.

How to talk to PWD

Check the person can hear you, ensuring any hearing aids are functioning well. Go to a less noisy area of the room if possible. Talk clearly and slowly in short sentences. Pause between sentences, giving the person time to understand the information. Let the person see your face as this will assist with lip reading and provide clues to what you are saying. The use of signs and mimicry, such as miming having something to eat or drink, wash or clean teeth, will also provide useful cues and help with overall understanding.

Age-related hearing loss, plus brain damage from the dementia, can interfere with both speech and hearing. Hence, it is useful to reduce noise within the environment because other sounds will make comprehension difficult because the loss of hearing cells will reduce people's abilities to filter out background noise.

In term of topics of conversation, it is important to recognise people's strengths and to remember that in addition to everyday social chit chat, their long-term memory will often be well preserved. Hence, talking about favourite hobbies, past jobs and achievements are all good ways to engage people. In our teaching programme we often suggest using the fundamental needs list as a template, therefore the best conversations will: be on a familiar topic, highlight their competencies, be fun and humorous, illustrate control and confidence, demonstrate they are liked and be non-threatening or demanding.

How to interact if physical contact is required

On occasions you may need to touch the PWD to assist with activities of daily living. They may not recognise you or think they do not need your help and thus they may be unhappy if you attempt to touch them (see Tanner, Chapter 8). In such circumstances it is often better to get initial contact via their consent. A common way to make a physical connection with someone you are not very familiar with is by offering a handshake. Once contact has been made the reassurance or assistance can be provided.

Teepa Snow suggests that when you are going to physically assist someone who is anxious or disorientated, contact should be made in three stages – visual, verbal and finally touch (see Thwaites, Chapter 7). Snow states that you should not touch someone, particularly when you need to assist them with intimate care, until you first get their attention through eye contact and a verbal exchange.

How to respond to difficult questions

On occasions PWD will ask difficult questions; the most problematic are often requests that are difficult to meet owing to the person being 'time shifted'. As discussed in the earlier section, the memory problems associated with time shifting mean that the person is no longer remembering the recent past but is drawing on memories from their LTM. Therefore the person may have forgotten: she has moved into care, her husband has died, she has retired, her children have grown up. Hence, the following questions are commonly heard from PWD:

- 'Can I leave the building, I want to get to home to cook my son's dinner?'

- 'The kids need collecting from school, can you open the door?'

- 'Can I go home, my mam is not well?'

- 'Can I get out of here and go to work?'

- 'What are all these people doing in my house?'

- 'Who is this person, she says she's my daughter?'

Sometimes these questions are ignored by carers, but if the PWD recognises her queries are either being avoided or remain unanswered, the questions may become repetitive. It is important for carers to acknowledge the query, so the person understands you have heard and understood. If the person is outwardly distressed or angry, it is also helpful to acknowledge that you have recognised their emotional state too.

In many situations it is helpful to use the RAM technique that we discussed in the previous chapters (Reduce the emotion, Assess the need, Meet the need). If you have used RAM and not been able to directly meet the person's need, as in the examples above, you should progress down the Needs Hierarchy (see Table 4.2).

Table 4.2: The Needs Hierarchy process

Steps	
1. Meet the *request* or *desire* directly	If one can give the person what she wants in an appropriate and safe manner, this should be done.
2. Substitute the *need* or validate the person's thinking	If one cannot meet the need directly then it may be possible to use a substitute. A substitute need may be appropriate because the person's specific request (e.g. to see deceased husband) may reflect a more general need (e.g. feeling lonely). The latter need is obviously more easily met via providing companionship. Alternatively, the person can be helped to talk about their original need to feel understood and accepted.

3. Distract/redirect from the current *need* to a new one	The carer should attempt to shift the person's need via distraction. It is hoped that through careful questioning and communication, the person will develop a new interest or desire, and forget the previous 'problematic' one.
4. Entering her reality: Meet the *need* via a therapeutic lie	Meet the need via the use of an 'untruth'. The contents of the deception should be wholly consistent with the person's biography. The Mental Health Foundation's recent report (2016) supports the use of untruths in such situations (see Chapter 6 for a full explanation of therapeutic lying).

Using the Needs Hierarchy, one first tries to discover what the person wants, such as a drink or to go to the toilet, and then simply fulfil the person's wish. In trying to determine the person's needs, we must look at the context: what the person is saying and their emotions in addition to the behaviour.

We may discover that the person's request is a means of getting something else. For example, a woman sitting in her room constantly shouting for her deceased husband may really want the company of others. Assisting her to go into the communal room may resolve the shouting.

If we cannot provide the person with her request, we must negotiate and see what can be done that will be an acceptable substitute. We may also try to validate the person's thinking and try to understand the reasons behind the current requests rather than addressing the content of their speech directly (Feil, 1993). If this does not work we may use distraction methods, and if all else fails we may have to employ a therapeutic lie as a last resort. The use of therapeutic lies will be discussed in more detail in Chapter 6. O'Connor and colleagues (2017) have provided a number of case studies on the use of the Needs Hierarchy in care home settings.

A recent survey on the phenomenon of time shifting has shown it to be very common in 24-hour care settings (Gibbons, Keddie and James, 2018) and carers are communicating with people who are time shifted on a daily basis. A detailed account of time shifting has been written by Mackenzie, Smith and James (2015), and a DVD providing case studies is also available (Mackenzie and James, 2010).

How to respond to repetitive questions

We have all experienced a phenomenon known as the Zeigarnik effect, which is the tendency for things we have planned to do to keep popping into our head until the action has been completed. This is sometimes also called a feeling of knowing. The Zeigarnik effect is very common in PWD because of their STM problems that we discussed earlier.

Hence, PWD cannot always remember whether they have either completed the task they had intended to do, or been given information about a question they had asked. The result of this problem can be repetitive questioning because they cannot remember the response given to them five minutes ago. Carers report this as a frustrating issue and describe it like listening to a 'broken repetitive record'.

Researchers have recognised the difficulties with repetitive questions (Snow, 2012; Hamdy et al., 2018a; Hamdy, et al., 2018b), and the following steps summarise the advice they give to deal with this issue:

1. Appreciate the questioning is often a manifestation of the PWD's concern about a particular issue.

2. Connect/reconnect to the person to show that you are attending fully to them. Ensure the person is feeling relaxed and secure.

3. Acknowledge the person's question/request. If you repeat the query, the person then knows you have understood it correctly (e.g. 'I see, you want to know where your daughter is').

4. Provide the most acceptable response/answer to the question (e.g. 'Your daughter has gone to the shops, she will be back at 2pm').

5. Respond using a number of modalities (auditory, visual and tactile) to reinforce information you are giving. For example, if someone is asking about the whereabouts of her purse, inform her that the purse is in her handbag, show her the purse in the bag and encourage her to touch and feel it.

6. Immediately, before the Zeigarnik effect arises again, try to redirect the person on to another topic. The new topic, with its new goal, must grab the person's attention such that they forget the original query ('Hi John, you're a big strong man, will you please help me put this box on the shelf?').

7. Ask the person for advice. Asking the person for advice is another strategy for getting her to focus on some other issue. However, ensure the person is not going to be overtaxed by your query.

A helpful series of case studies on how to deal with repetitive questions have been published by Hamdy and colleagues (2018a; 2018b). Their case studies indicate that the phenomenon is highly frustrating for carers, but it is important for the carer to remain calm because emotional reactions can increase the frequency of the questions. Hamdy and colleagues describe the sorts of topics that are likely to help redirect the PWD, and these areas map well with our own fundamental needs list:

- Engage the person in conversations that make her feel needed, wanted, loved and secure.

- Talk about recreational activities she enjoys.

- Enlist the person's help in activities that she thinks she's still competent to do (e.g. sort items into piles, sweep the floor, clear the table).

STOP START SCENARIOS FOR BEHAVIOURS THAT CHALLENGE (BTC)

Once a problem behaviour (BtC) has occurred it will then require an interaction in the form of an intervention to resolve the difficulty and minimise the risk. In such scenarios, we are often required to act persuasively to get the PWD to either stop some problematic behaviour or to start a behaviour aimed at enhancing the person's wellbeing.

These interactions are referred to as 'Stop Start Scenarios' (SSS) (James and Hope, 2013) and we believe that the essence of dealing well with BtC is the ability to intervene appropriately with SSS. The common SSS include:

- Stop: Preventing someone leaving the building, hitting out, shouting, going into someone's room.

- Start: Assisting someone to get up in the morning, helping someone go to the toilet, helping someone engage in self-care activities, encouraging someone to take medication, asking someone to go to bed, asking someone to have a wash.

We suggest that training to communicate effectively around these common daily activities is essential to delivering good dementia care. Furthermore, knowing these sorts of activities are likely to be the triggers for BtC, we are in a good position to develop skills for such interactions.

INTERVENTIONS WHEN SOMEONE IS DISTRESSED OR CHALLENGING

When dealing with situations when someone is already engaging in a BtC, it is often the carer's role to de-escalate the situation, calm the person and deal with any potential risk.

Research suggests that there are number of things *not* to do in order not to inflame the situation, and we already have seen the Verbal Judo technique in Chapter 3 that addresses some of these issues. There are two other useful approaches in this area: the first is based on training supported by the American Veteran's Association (Flaherty, 2015), which we have termed DATA, and the other is called BANGS (Macaulay, 2015). We examine these methods below:

DATA (aka T-A-DA method)

The letters DATA spell out the three key approaches suggested by Flaherty (2015) to deal with BtC – Don't Agitate, Tolerate, Anticipate:

Don't Agitate (DA)

If one sees a resident undressing in a communal room, approach her calmly and guide her to a more private area, rather than shouting 'Stop' and rushing towards her.

Tolerate and accept (T)

When one witnesses an unusual behaviour, one should ask whether it requires any kind of immediate intervention. Are there any immediate risks to the person or others? If there are no concerns, one may be able to simply tolerate the actions.

Anticipate (A)

Residents have regular patterns to their behaviours (time of day, triggers). If one can anticipate when a behaviour is likely to happen, one can intervene in a way prior to any problems emerging. For example, if John always gets upset after his wife leaves the home, spending a few minutes with him until he forgets she's left may reduce his desire to leave the care facility.

BANGS

When communicating with PWD there can be situations where the most appropriate action is to accept their perspectives, even if their views are inconsistent with reality (e.g. a person living with dementia incorrectly accusing her daughter of taking her purse). Susan Macaulay, a family carer, developed the acronym BANGS to describe such an 'acceptance' method (Macaulay, 2015). BANGS highlights the following six features.

Breathe

When you recognise that a confrontation is likely to arise in which you will be required to intervene, before doing anything else take time to 'centre' yourself. A good way of centring yourself is to stop and take a deep breath. This technique is also used by many athletes just before doing something important, such as taking a penalty kick in football.

Assess, accept and agree

Try to make a logical assessment of the current situation, and attempt to understand what is going on. Listen to what the person is saying and try to clarify the situation. If there is no immediate danger for the person or others, be prepared to accept the person's statements and her views wholeheartedly. Positively agree with the person's view, confirming that she is correct and thereby validating her perspective and making her feel good.

Never argue

Macaulay says 'never, never argue!' She asks carers who get into lots of confrontations an important question: 'Would you rather be happy or right?'

Go and let go

The 'go' element refers to 'going with the flow' of the person living with dementia, and not letting the carer's ego get in the way. In terms of the latter, the carer must be prepared to 'let go' of being correct and not try to direct the person. The 'go' also refers to the fact that once people are no longer feeling agitated they can shift their concentration onto a different topic.

Say sorry

To complete the protocol it is necessary to apologise. By saying sorry the episode is ended and PWD are likely to feel their needs have been met, so potential resentment has been dissipated. Hence, it should be a proper sorry that is conveyed in terms of both body language and tone of voice.

BANGS is a useful technique to use in situations where PWD are expressing an opinion or making an accusation, such as a person claiming she is still working or misidentifing you as someone else.

Case study using BANGS: Mother accusing son of stealing her handbag

A son notices that his mother is searching for her handbag and he recognises that if she does not find it in the next minute, she will accuse him of having stolen it. He then takes a deep breath (B) in preparation to deal with his mother's accusations. A minute later...

Mother: What have you done with my handbag? I put it here a few minutes ago. Where is it?

Son (assesses the situation and recognises that it is safe to accept (A) the blame for the handbag, and so he does): I must have moved it by mistake when I was tidying things up. Let me help you search.

Note that he does not attempt to argue, despite him being blameless (never argue, N).

Mother: You shouldn't touch my stuff. It's got my money in it. You're so stupid sometimes.

She bosses him around, telling him where to search. He does not get upset, but merely goes with the flow (G).

Eventually, they find the handbag. Nevertheless, mother is still agitated, therefore the son apologises.

Son: I am really glad you've got your handbag back and I am really sorry to have caused such a fuss. I'll be more careful in the future, sorry Mum.

This is the sorry (S) that attempts to resolve the issue for the PWD and deal with any residual frustration.

SUMMARY

The brain is like the central control room of a giant rail system, with traffic going back and forth all the time to all areas of the network. Most of the system runs automatically, but occasionally a controller has to make a decision or deal with an error or problem. However, if the rail organisation started losing its controllers, and could no longer respond to errors, it would not take too long before the whole network failed.

When this analogy is applied to dementia, we can see that dementia is a disease of the whole body and not just related to poor memory or decision-making. The brain cells (like the controllers) are responsible for running and coordinating a complex network. In this chapter we have illustrated some of the sensory and physical changes that occur alongside the intellectual difficulties. Indeed, it is vital for carers to recognise that the way they approach, talk and touch PWD requires some careful thought and empathy. During communication we should ensure PWD feel safe, valued, pain free and comfortable, respected and relevant. When all these needs are fulfilled it is less likely that the person will engage in BtC.

The chapter has also provided specific techniques such as the Needs Hierarchy, DATA and BANGS, which can help structure one's communication and interaction skills.

Chapter Five

Activities of Daily Living (ADL) and Levels of Functioning: Spokes

In Chapter 5 we focus on how to communicate and interact with PWD during activities such as intimate care tasks and daily chores. If the appropriate levels of support are not given by carers during activities, the person may feel frustrated, patronised or angry, which can result in BtC.

We also give guidance on how to adapt communication styles to meet the needs of PWD, considering the level at which the person can undertake tasks for themselves.

LEVELS OF FUNCTIONING AND RAM

In relation to RAM the two features that should be emphasised are: (i) how to relate sensitively to people who are receiving help with intimate care tasks; and (ii) how to meet the needs of people who lack insight into their own needs and difficulties.

Relating to people during ADL

Supporting people during activities of daily living (ADL) requires entry to the PWD's personal space and often having to touch them. This places a demand on the relationship and requires the carer, even when he knows the person well, to reconnect and reintroduce himself. The latter helps prepare the PWD for any kind of intimate touch that may occur.

In this context we discuss the work of Teepa Snow (Hand under Hand techniques, HuH™, see Thwaites, Chapter 7) as an example of effective connecting. This is a supportive handhold where your hand is moved under the person's hand and cradles it. This permits the person to feel supported and allows the carer to be able to use their free fingers to assist with washing, feeding and other hygiene activities. The advantage of the technique is that whenever you are engaging in the activity, the simultaneous movement of the PWD's hand and arm often gives them the impression they are doing activities for themselves. This reduces potential resistance when staff are giving assistance with intimate care activities.

Meeting the needs of people with poor insight

Confrontations can sometimes occur when PWD fail to recognise they have a need that must be fulfilled regarding their personal care or safety. For example, a person may refuse medication, insist he is still capable of driving, or fail to recognise his clothes are soiled. In such situations the conflict is a result of clashing needs: the need of the carer/organisation to deliver appropriate care versus the needs of the individual in relation to independence, control and dignity. In this section, we are particularly focused on aligning these sets of needs with respect to personal care issues.

WHAT IS MEANINGFUL ACTIVITY?

Humans have an innate desire to have a purpose and meaning in life (Wilcock, 1993). Meaningful days matter to all people and this is also true for someone who is living with dementia. Engaging in meaningful activity can fulfil many of the fundamental needs of PWD as has been discussed previously.

According to Ranka and Chapparo (1997), there are four categories of activity that help human beings feel valued, purposeful and provide a sense of dignity and belonging (Table 5.1), and these are equally relevant for people with or without cognitive impairment. Evidence suggests there is a clear link between a lack of meaningful occupation and engagement and BtC.

Table 5.1: Categories of activity

1. Work	This is a very important life experience that gives a person the sense of making a difference. When we work we learn that what we do is of value to others as well as ourselves. This is critical in creating a sense of wellbeing and continued self-esteem.
2. Leisure	Activities we do because they are fun, make us feel good or give us joy. These activities can be either passive or active and they tend to improve both a person's mood and energy levels.
3. Self-care	Taking care of ourselves is about the big and the little things in our personal 'world of needs'. This includes personal care tasks and attention to our body, our mind, our environment, our business, and even how we move ourselves from place to place.

cont.

4. Rest and restoration	This is one that we don't often think of as an activity but is a part of how we fill our day. This is especially important to be aware of when someone is experiencing brain change. Rest not only includes our sleep but also incorporates a period of time that a person may need to either be alone or with others, a time that helps a person to recharge or restore themselves.

It can be challenging to facilitate these activities because PWD often do not have the same level of skills or access to previous occupational roles and interests. We need to understand the impact of the cognitive impairment on an individual's ability to support himself to engage in meaningful occupations. This will then help us to ensure that we support individuals in the right way, facilitating them to engage in the things which bring meaning and pleasure to their lives.

When supporting people's ADL there may arise a conflict of needs: the needs of the PWD versus the needs associated with his best interests versus organisational needs. For example, prior to entering a care home Joe may have always slept late and gone to bed after midnight. Such a pattern, however, may not fit well with a care home's rather rigid nighttime policy. Under the guise of health and safety legislation, the management may insist that everyone is in bed by 10pm.

'JUST RIGHT CHALLENGE'

A 'just right challenge' is a very careful balance between the challenge of the task and the skills of the person in order to provide a positive experience. We need to support the person just enough for them to complete the task. Too little might lead to failure, too much would deskill the person. If the balance is not established this may lead to frustration, increased anxiety and confusion.

Evidence suggests that many staff do not receive sufficient training in assisting with ADL. This is a serious problem as we know that BtC frequently occur around tasks to do with delivering intimate care.

INTRODUCTION TO THE POOL ACTIVITY LEVEL (PAL) INSTRUMENT

A helpful framework for guiding carers about what level of support they need to provide during ADL is the Pool Activity Level (PAL) Instrument, (Pool, 2012). The PAL Instrument outlines a four-stage framework to help carers deliver care at the correct level. It describes people's abilities in terms of Planned, Exploratory, Sensory and Reflex levels. The principles underlying the instrument are:

- All people with cognitive impairment have some abilities.

- A person's potential can be reached if an activity/task is presented in a way which the person can engage.

- The role of the carer is 'to create a just right environment' so that the PWD can participate in an activity.

- A person is more likely to engage with the activity if it has personal significance, related to their life history and personal preference.

From our perspective we are particularly interested in assessing how we continue to meet people's fundamental needs during the progression through the levels/stages of dementia (Figure 5.1).

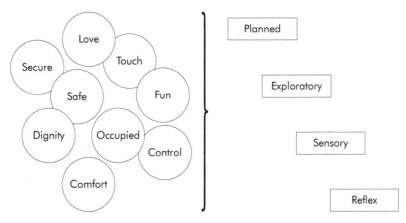

Figure 5.1: Matching fundamental needs with level of dementia

In the PAL Instrument each of the levels represent stages of abilities the person will pass through as the disease progresses from Planned towards Reflex.

Planned

Someone operating at this level will have a mild dementia, therefore a carer's role is often to maximise independence and optimise use of any existing skills. One of the person's main strengths is his continued ability to plan tasks, although he may struggle to carry out complex activities. Although at this stage people may be able to plan, they often struggle to problem solve situations. When communicating, carers will need to keep sentences short, factual and simple, avoiding using words like 'and' or 'but', which tend to link two sentences together making them complex.

Exploratory

At this level the person likes to be active and occupied. People often explore their environment, sometimes because of poor orientation and memory difficulties. They can carry out familiar activities, if the tasks involve relatively simple actions and are being carried out in familiar surroundings. The person may not be overly interested in the outcome of an action and may seem more focused on being active. If carers want to help the person to do something, they may need to break the activity into manageable chunks.

Sensory

The person is more interested in feeling and experiencing sensations rather than carrying out tasks. They will often touch, feel and smell things, and engage in lots of non-purposeful walking. They may be guided to carry out single-step activities such as sweeping or winding wool. The person may be cued into activities using mime and copying tasks.

Reflex

This level occurs at the most severe stage of the dementia process and the person may not be very aware of their surroundings or even his own body. He is living in a state where movement is a reflex response to a stimulus. Carers need to use direct sensory stimulation but must be careful because multiple stimuli can cause distress. Communication is mainly via the use of facial expression and a warm and reassuring tone, and appropriate volume is important (see Ellis and Astell, Chapter 9).

Alignment of carer skills with the PAL Instrument

There are some basic principles that can be considered for all PWD with respect to ADL:

- *Assessing – Is the person ready?* Undertaking personal care activities is a common source of anxiety for PWD. Therefore, prior to attempting to assist with any form of ADL, assess whether the PWD is ready to undertake the task. If the person is agitated, the ADL may need to be postponed until later.

- *Connect/Reconnect.* Always pay attention to connecting well with the person before any care activity. The first step is to gain their attention through vision; second, add in verbal communication, at the right level for the person; and lastly touch (Snow, 2012; Thwaites, Chapter 7). Touch is the most invasive form of connection and the carer should not touch the person unless a good connection has been first made via the first two steps.

- *HuH™.* The Hand under Hand (Snow, 2012) technique is designed to offer assistance and memory cueing in a supportive and collaborative approach, as described previously. HuH™ is most appropriate for people in the sensory and reflex stages of PAL.

- *Initiation.* In the later stages of dementia, people will start to struggle to initiate and activate action memories, even automatic ones, and in these circumstances, they may need help in activating. Sometimes full assistance with the activity may be required.

By using PAL we can enhance our caregiving skills. It allows us to better tailor our interventions in relation to people's strengths, helping us to adjust our goals and expectations.

The following three case studies (Mary, Fred and Alice) show how PWD with different PAL levels can be supported during ADL. In each case the approximate level on the PAL Instrument will be indicated, however the main emphasis is to illustrate the fact that our approach needs to adapt according to the person. Many of the features relating to dementia that were presented in the previous chapters are important if we want to tailor our approach to the individual (memory, sensory changes, type of dementia).

Case study: Mary – early stages of dementia (PAL Exploratory)

Mary:

- is not aware that she needs support with any personal care tasks and thinks that she is still routinely doing these things for herself

- sometimes repeats tasks or steps of tasks over and over

- can get sequencing mixed up and misses steps out – puts clothes on in wrong order

- will use things that are out on view but will not look in cupboards or drawers

- can start off doing something but gets distracted and forgets the task at hand

- likes to be in control and may resist or refuse help when needed

- has fluctuating memory, orientation and way-finding abilities; better on some occasions than others

- likes to be busy and to do things

- can have difficulty understanding complicated instructions or explanations, especially when she is tired or upset

- may not always be able to find the words for things she wants to say.

Case study: Fred – moderate stages of dementia (PAL Sensory)

Fred:

- lacks safety awareness

- likes to explore with his hands and touch things as he goes

- can get over-stimulated, especially as the day goes on

- has no awareness of others needs and may invade others' space

- is often unable to make his needs known

- may not understand why/what care-givers are doing

- does not like being helped or touched during personal care

- likes to do things that are one-step and repetitive

- needs one step at a time instructions

- can use social chit chat that is very superficial – can unintentionally trick people into thinking he is more cognitively aware than he is

- has little understanding of what is said to him, especially when he is anxious or distressed

- understands the rhythm of speech and so will get a lot of meaning from the para-verbals (i.e. the way we say things).

Case study: Alice – later stages of dementia (PAL Sensory/Reflex)

Alice:

- has difficulty processing/coping with more than one sensation at a time

- is unable to understand what is said to her, which means she cannot benefit from reassurance, instructions or explanations at all. This means that when staff are supporting her with personal care, she misunderstands their intentions and reacts by trying to protect herself from what she perceives as harm

- has some social chit chat, but on the whole what she says is unintelligible

- can still sing

- is unable to communicate or recognise her internal bodily cues (physical or emotional needs)

- has lost motor control of eye, fingers, mouth and feet

- has changes in her visual field and appears not to notice things to the side of her, attending more to what is lower down and directly in front of her.

Applying the PAL Instrument principles to assistance with bathing

We will now examine using the PAL Instrument with particular ADL to demonstrate the adjustments that may be required across the PAL levels. Having a bath is a very intimate experience and people can find it embarrassing and/or threatening when someone else is watching and assisting. Being seen naked is a particular problem and was the most upsetting item mentioned by care workers when they were asked, what they would fear most if they needed to go into 24 hour care (James *et al.*, 2016).

Some people may feel isolated and become anxious if they are left on their own and may want their carer to stay with them while they are washing. However, problems can occur if the carer is unfamiliar or a member of the opposite sex, or focuses too much on the task, and not enough on the person.

Being nude when others have their clothes on can be uncomfortable. Avoiding complete nudity and keeping the time when the person is fully naked to a minimum may reduce possible embarrassment. Some people can enter the bath clothed by using a light cotton dressing gown, but once clothes are wet they often choose to de-robe themselves. It is not necessary to wash the whole body on each occasion and it may be better to wash a different part of the body thoroughly every day.

It is helpful for the PWD to participate in the bathing exercise and they can hold the soap or sponge. This is a useful technique for people who sometimes become sexually disinhibited and try to grab their carers.

Washing hair can be particularly difficult due to physical difficulties such as arthritis, therefore this may be done at a different time from the rest of bathing. Avoid the use of a shampoo, which will cause stinging if it gets into the person's eyes, or use a dry shampoo that can clean the hair without using water.

Check the water temperature and level, which should ideally be low when the person first gets in and can be topped up later. To assist the person to judge depth, place a coloured non-slip mat at the bottom of the bath. Some people find the rush of water from an overhead shower frightening or disorienting, therefore a hand-held shower may work better. People may also find it scary stepping into water due to problems with depth perception.

We will need to adapt the skills listed above to meet the needs of people with different levels of functional abilities, as can be seen in the case studies of Mary, Fred and Alice.

Case study: Supporting Mary with bathing – early stages of dementia (PAL Exploratory)

- Broaching the subject of having a bath will be the most difficult thing with Mary because she thinks she has just had one. You may need to acknowledge that she has had a bath recently but would she like a soak and some pampering – offer and be careful not to point out anything negative.

- Find out what her usual routine used to be – did she bathe morning or evening or a particular day of the week?

- Break down the task into manageable chunks: suggest that Mary fills the bath, then when that is accomplished suggest that she gathers together items such as soap, shampoo, a flannel, and towels – do 'with' her rather than 'to' her.

- When Mary is in the bath, suggest that she soaps and rinses her upper body, and when that is accomplished, then suggest that she soaps and rinses her lower body.

- Ensure that all items needed are on view and that containers are clearly labelled.

- It is about Mary doing as much for herself as possible, and feeling she is in control.

Case study: Supporting Fred with bathing – moderate stages of dementia (PAL Sensory)

- Fred will need an environmental cue to help him understand what is going to happen, so prepare the bathroom and run the bath water for him.

- Make the bathroom warm.

- He will need one-step-at-a-time simple directions: 'rub the soap on the cloth, rub your arm, rinse your arm, rub your chest, rinse your chest'.

- Alongside the directions you will need to demonstrate by an action what you want Fred to do and offer him the item he needs to use.

- He is less embarrassed with female carers as he associates females with caring for him, and his wife used to wash his hair for him in the bath (but some men prefer another male).

- He needs a towel for modesty to reduce his distress and embarrassment – let him leave this on even when in the water – he will usually remove it once it is wet.

- Make sure there are as few staff as possible – have others on stand-by outside if needed.

- Fred may need us to use HuH™ guidance.

Case study: Supporting Alice with bathing – later stages of dementia (PAL Sensory/Reflex)

- Prepare the bathroom and run the bath water for Alice; put in scented bath products that are very familiar to her and are her favourites.

- Ensure that the bathroom is warm.

- Do not touch her until you have first got verbal and visual attention, or she will get startled.

- Use HuH™ to make sure touch feels less invasive.

- Use firm, slow massaging movements when soaping and rinsing Alice.

- Singing or humming a tune together may help to connect and provide rhythm for the task.

- Wrap Alice securely in a warm towel when she is out of the bath.

Applying the PAL Instrument to improve the mealtime experience

Mealtimes can be an enjoyable experience for some but can also be a time of great stress and distress for others. Supporting the nutritional intake of PWD is important and adequate food and fluid intake is vital in maintaining health and wellbeing. Once a person's level of function has been identified, care-givers can use this information to help plan the mealtime experience.

Planned level

People functioning on a planned level should be able to identify that they are hungry. They can be encouraged to be involved in the setting up of the dining room, helping to set the table and select crockery and cutlery. He will be able to use a knife and fork appropriately. Condiments can be displayed on the table, and at this stage should not cause too much distraction. A person at planned level has good communication skills, so encourage them to sit with people of similar level. He will prefer to sit in their usual place. The person will be able to choose what they want to eat and read a menu if provided.

Exploratory level

At this level people will recognise they are hungry but may forget when they last ate. They will be able to be involved in the setting up of the dining table with cutlery and crockery. He will use a spoon, but a fork and knife may be too taxing, and he may require food to be cut. A pictorial menu can support the person to make independent choices about what they want to eat. They will be able to sit with others and enjoy each other's company.

Sensory level

At the sensory level people may not recognise when they are hungry, nor be able to recall what, and when, they last ate. The dining table will need to be set up prior to the person sitting down at the table; placemats will provide visual cues and all unnecessary items such as condiments should be removed to avoid distraction. A carer will need to be on hand to encourage the person to remain seated and attend to their meal. Noise and other potential distractions should be reduced within the dining area. Contrasting coloured crockery should be used to help with visual difficulties. The person may be able to choose his meal from a pictorial menu board, however, it is better to limit the choices to two items. Finger food may need to be offered, and/or HuH™ guidance can be used to start the action of bringing food to the mouth.

Reflex level

At this level people may not recognise hunger or be able to communicate the need for food. People may require the full support of one carer and the person may eat better in their own room or in a quiet area. Visual prompts are very helpful and showing two plates of food will facilitate decisions about choice. The dining table should be set up in advance and condiments should be removed. Contrasting crockery should be used, the person may prefer finger foods; otherwise HuH™ techniques can be used.

A helpful case study provides further guidance on meal times (Hamdy et al., 2018c). This example illustrates the difficulties associated with someone eating at a restaurant, and the manner in which distractions can lead to BtC in someone with a frontotemporal dementia.

Applying the PAL Instrument to assist with using the toilet

Supporting PWD to remain independent with using the toilet should be a key priority. Unfortunately too often we see this skill can be lost due to lack of appropriate support of the person (Stokes, 2006). By identifying a person's level of functioning and then planning the assistance required, we will help PWD to retain continence skills for longer.

Planned level

At a planned level the person should be able to use the toilet independently and will need assistance only when problems arise. The person is able to locate the toilet within their local environment. However, toilets should be well signposted as the person may struggle in unfamiliar environments. He should be independent with transfers when no other physical conditions exist and should be able to adjust his clothing and manage underwear; minimal assistance and/or prompts may be needed. A sign to prompt the person to remember to wash hands would be useful.

Exploratory level

A person functioning at an exploratory level should be able to use the toilet independently but will require assistance at times when problems arise. Toilets need to be well signposted and there needs to be directions around the building guiding to the nearest toilet. The person may require prompts to use the toilet and if he has an en-suite, one should leave the door open so that the person can see the toilet. They should be able to transfer independently providing there are no other physical difficulties. The person may need to wear manageable clothes because it can be difficult for him to manage underwear, tights and zipped or buttoned trousers. He may need a prompt to use toilet roll to clean himself, but if handed toilet roll he should be able to complete this task independently.

Sensory level

At a sensory level a person's ability to recognise and communicate a need for the toilet fluctuates. Carers should be aware of this and observe for when he seems to be searching or looks uncomfortable. The person may need to be prompted to use the toilet and will need to be accompanied to the toilet; he may benefit from a toilet scheduling. The person may not recognise a toilet so will need to be prompted. He will most likely need assistance and guidance to sit down. They may have difficulty backing up to sit on the toilet, as walking backward can become difficult. He will need assistance to remove clothing and underwear; he may be able to follow single-step instructions to assist. If the toilet roll is easily visible and of a domestic style, he will be able to do most of the steps for himself; carers will need to be on hand to ensure personal hygiene is maintained. Simple single-step instructions are needed, and the person may need physical support to wash hands.

Reflex level

A person functioning at reflex level may not recognise his own bodily cues so carers should look for cues and signs (e.g. if the person is agitated, fidgeting or tugging on clothing, or touching the genital area). The person should be accompanied to the toilet, and may not recognise a toilet pan and so will need to be guided. He may require a reminder of why he is on the toilet once there. Otherwise he may not stay long enough to complete the task. He will most likely require assistance and guidance to sit down/stand up from the toilet; HuH™ can be used to assist with undressing. The person will also be reliant upon carers to attend to intimate personal care and hand hygiene.

In the past we have conducted studies with care staff which have shown that there are many anxieties associated with using toilets, particularly public toilets (James *et al.*, 2007). Such projects have shown that many of the general population avoid using toilets outside of the home, or have unusual hygienic rituals when required to use public toilets (e.g. hovering over the bowl, or placing a nest of paper on the top of the seat). Hence, imagine the anxieties that PWD may experience when required to use an unfamiliar toilet in the company of someone else! It is not hard to envisage why continence difficulties might start to arise.

SUMMARY

Staff are often supporting people to undertake personal hygiene activities. Owing to the intimate nature and potential invasiveness surrounding activities of daily living, these activities are often triggers to BtC. In order to minimise distress and agitation, this chapter has highlighted the hands-on carer skills required to manage and navigate daily living in a sensitive, dignified and empathic manner. The chapter has introduced the PAL Instrument as a tool for adapting the amount of assistance provided by carers to match the skill levels of the PWD.

Chapter Six
....

Formulation-Led Approaches: Rim

In this chapter we will learn about complex assessments, formulations and formulation-led interventions. The concept of the Needs Hierarchy (see also Chapter 4, Table 4.2), including therapeutic lies, will be discussed. We generally see aspects of the rim as being used with people displaying either high-risk behaviours or chronic BtC that have not responded well to previous strategies. As such, working at this level is more resource intensive and requires a higher range of skills.

The use of RAM (Reduce the emotion, Assess the need, Meet the need) is critical in how we deliver the approach in this section. However, the features of RAM differ slightly. We need to spend a lot more time on:

- the Assessment of need, as it involves the development of a formulation

- being clear how to Meet the need, which we do through the writing of a care plan.

TREATMENTS FOR DIFFICULT TO RESOLVE BTC

In the past BtC were regarded as a common feature or symptom of dementia. Since we did not have a treatment for dementia, we tried to control the unwanted behaviours, and this was usually done via tranquilisers and sedatives. Unfortunately, because the behaviours were not true symptoms, the drugs were often ineffective (Banerjee, 2009). While there is a very important role for medication in the treatment of BtC, over the last 10 years we have also learned a lot more about medication's highly problematic side-effects. The potential role for medication is recognised, but now we have a better understanding of the causes of BtC, medications are used alongside other non-drug strategies. Figure 6.1 outlines some of the traditional treatment strategies.

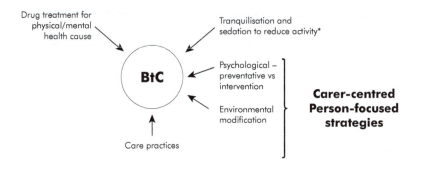

* In situations where the behaviours displayed pose a threat to either the person or people in her environment, emergency actions will be required. This may include the immediate use of tranquilising/sedating medication. However, owing to the highly problematic side-effects and ethical difficulties associated with these types of interventions, it is recommended that in the majority of situations the carer-centred, person-focused strategies are trialled first (NICE, 2018).

Figure 6.1: Traditional treatment strategies

Antipsychotic medication

First-generation antipsychotic drugs, known as typical antipsychotics, were discovered in the 1950s to reduce psychotic experiences such as paranoid thoughts and hallucinations. More recent types of antipsychotics (i.e. second-generation, atypicals) are well known for having a tranquilising effect. They are believed to be effective in 20 to 30 per cent of cases of BtC (Banerjee, 2009), but their tranquilising effects are generic, making the person less interested in self-care tasks, thereby de-skilling the individual. Further, any stress or distress underpinning the BtC is not dealt with directly, rather the symptoms associated with the distress are merely dampened down (James and Jackman, 2017).

In the absence of any more suitable medication, antipsychotics have been used routinely to treat BtC. However, it is widely recognised that they are not particularly effective with PWD and they often have highly problematic side-effects. This has led to guidelines which suggest that antipsychotics should be:

- used only as an initial step if there is an immediate danger to the PWD or someone in the vicinity (NICE, 2018)

- used after an initial trial of an environmental or person-centred approach

- given for a short period and then assessed every 12 weeks in terms of benefits and side-effects

- administered at a low dose and withdrawn as soon as possible

- used with great caution with certain types of dementia such as dementia with Lewy bodies (DLB) because of potentially fatal consequences.

Benzodiazepines such as diazepam and lorazepam, which can cause sedation, must also be used with great care in PWD. Their use is frequently associated with confusion and falls.

Prescribing in this area has always been difficult, which is in part due to the slower metabolising abilities of older people, leading to higher degrees of toxicity at lower doses. However, most of the problematic side-effects are due to the powerful generic impact of some of these drugs on people's bodies. Polypharmacy is also a concern, with many older people taking numerous different medications for various physical and mental health conditions (Royal College of Psychiatrists, 2011; Patterson et al., 2012).

In our modern approach to BtC, dementia is no longer seen as the first and most important cause, it is now seen as only one of many potential causes of the difficult behaviour. The following section outlines the common causes and examines an up-to-date approach to BtC. You will notice that good communication plays a key role in non-drug treatments of BtC.

UNMET NEEDS: BTC OCCURRING DUE TO NEEDS NOT BEING MET

For PWD, there tends to be eight common areas where needs may go unmet, and consequently BtC may emerge (see Table 6.1).

Table 6.1: Areas associated with unmet needs and causes of BtC

Areas	Factors influencing needs and behaviour	Methods of managing/treating factors
Lack of physical comfort	The nature and management of the physical problems will determine person's needs: Delirium Pain (including dental) Constipation Arthritis Sensory problems	PINCH ME check for delirium (Pain, Infection, Nutrition, Constipation, Hydration, Medication, Environment) Physical checks and appropriate physical treatments

Feeling unsafe	Feelings of being unsafe physically and psychologically, worries and concerns about where you are, and what is going to happen next	Providing a sense of safety by promoting structure and routine within the setting, making the environment more predictable. Ensuring the PWD does not feel vulnerable
Lack of sense of belonging/love	Feeling lonely, unwanted and not part of the group	Promoting a sense of feeling worthwhile and wanted. Encouraging participation in group activities
Lack of respect/ being taken advantage of	Feeling of being disrespected and treated unjustly	Ensuring the person feels her rights are upheld and opinion taken into account
Lack of control of environment	Environmental layout may not be 'dementia friendly' leading to needs emerging. Carer interactions and ability to meet or not meet the PWD's needs	Improve orientation through altering layout. Improve communication skills to increase wellbeing and reduce unnecessary confrontation
Lack of positive touch	Lack of visit from family. Isolating herself due to loneliness or depression	Appropriate massage. Touching person at other times to provide comfort rather than as part of a task
Lack of opportunity to do things and have fun	Lack of meaningful activity. Sense of boredom	Provide opportunities to engage with surroundings and others to relieve boredom. Engage PWD in activities which they used to like and still may retain some skills in

This table highlights several important issues:

- Unmet needs may arise from either one single factor (e.g. infection) or a combination of factors (e.g. infection, over-medication, unsuitable environment, feeling disrespected).

- Even if the causes are similar, two people may present very differently (e.g. if two people have Alzheimer's disease and both are in pain, one person may constantly shout while the other may hit out).

- The complexity of any treatment will depend on the number of potential areas involved and the type of behaviour displayed, such as verbal aggression or sexual disinhibition.

- On occasions treatments can be quick and simple, while at other times we need an in-depth assessment and maybe the help of a specialist team.

The 'Methods of managing' column of Table 6.1 highlights that basic carer's actions (support and interaction) are a very common management strategy when attempting to meet people's needs. In such cases the carers are required to understand a person's unmet need and then adjust their own communication and interactions accordingly.

FORMULATION-LED INTERVENTIONS: COMPREHENSIVE ASSESSMENTS TO IDENTIFY AND MEET PWD'S NEEDS

The following formulation-led approaches are viewed as the best approaches for the treatment of persistent BtC (James and Moniz-Cook, 2018; Holle *et al.*, 2016). They typically seek to investigate all the features outlined in Table 6.1 to ensure the potential unmet needs are addressed. We have learnt that if carers have a better understanding of the reason behind the behaviours, they will try to change their ways of working to resolve them. All problem behaviours are episodic; they all have patterns and formulation-led approaches are designed to identify such patterns. Indeed, the whole point of undertaking a formulation is to find and disrupt the repetitive dysfunctional patterns and their triggers.

Over the years we have worked closely with care staff to see what information is useful for them to collect to better understand BtC. The needs outlined in Table 6.1 were a guide for this, but when we discussed this with the staff we found they preferred to identify the key needs from information they had available in the PWD's files and personal records within the care home (see Figure 6.2). By putting together the information contained in Figure 6.2 staff felt they could identify the relevant unmet need(s).

In BtC, there are several different types of formulations used to try to explain this behaviour (Holle *et al.*, 2016). They all have the same aims, which include looking at possible causes and obtaining information about each of the causes to see if they may explain the PWD's needs and behaviour.

In the North East of England one of the most frequently used formulations is the Newcastle Framework (James, 1999, see Figure 6.3). This framework includes an eight- to 12-week collaborative inter-vention program, comprised of the following four phases: background assessment, assessment of triggers of BtC, information sharing session, interventions.

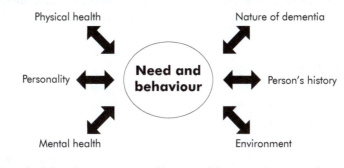

Each of these features is a possible cause of the BtC and a potential target for treatment if found to be a cause

Figure 6.2: Six features of unmet needs and BtC

Phase 1: Background assessment of person's BtC

Information is gathered about the person's background including their life story and physical and mental health from friends, family, care-givers and from case files and relevant databases. The assessment material is gathered by a member of a specialist BtC team (e.g. the Behaviour Support Team) with the assistance of the person's key worker.

Phase 2: Assessment of triggers of BtC

Information is collected about events or situations which are eliciting the behaviours. This is done through discussion and completion of behavioural charts (see later section). These charts provide detailed information regarding each 'problem' behaviour and the staff's reactions to them.

Phase 3: Information Sharing Session (ISS, aka Formulation Session)

A member of the Behaviour Support Team collates the information gathered above and sets up a meeting (Information Sharing Session, ISS) with the people involved in the person's care. This includes staff, family and other professionals, and the aim is to develop a shared understanding of why the person is displaying the various behaviours. Typically, such sessions change the carers from being problem-focused to solution-focused in their thinking. This is done by increasing empathy and improving understanding of the person's behaviours. A tangible product of this session is a summary of all the information that has been collected about the person in the form of a single A4 sheet, called the Newcastle Framework. Figure 6.3 presents a simplified version of the Newcastle Framework.

Phase 4: Interventions

Interventions are based on the group's suggestions from the ISS meeting, then developed and refined within a care plan (see later section). Ongoing support is provided for four weeks by the clinician from the Behaviour Support Team to ensure appropriate implementation of the treatment strategies. Some of the non-drug interventions are discussed later in this chapter. Tweaking of the care plans are undertaken where necessary.

Case study: Illustrating Michael's formulation

Aged 79, Michael was referred to the Behaviour Support Team for displaying extreme aggression. The staff were so frightened of him that they rushed all his ADL and rarely spoke to him. He spent a lot of time alone in his room, except when family visited. He was never aggressive towards his family. The staff had no explanation for his behaviour, although they incorrectly said, 'it is probably because he has Lewy body dementia'.

From the ISS meeting Michael's formulation was completed, which summarised key areas and outlined some potential causal factors regarding his aggression. This summary gave an explanatory story, as follows:

> Michael typically got out of the bed during the night to go to the toilet and would often fall on his way to the bathroom, falling on his left side. The falls were due to several reasons including: the strange arrangement of the bed within the room, his poor mobility, poor lighting and his DLB. Owing to his dementia, by morning he would forget what had happened. However, when he awoke he would experience pain and notice bruises on his body. He interpreted this as being beaten up during the night while he was defenceless in bed. This made him extremely angry and he wanted to get his revenge. He targeted the male staff in particular because he did not believe a woman could overpower him.

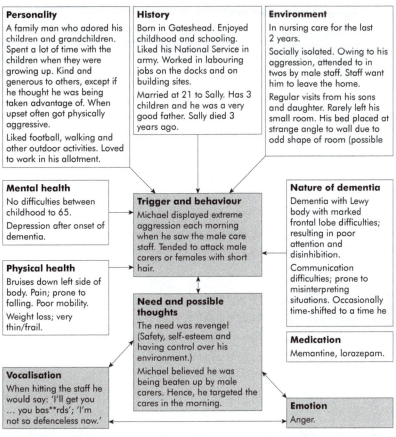

Personality
A family man who adored his children and grandchildren. Spent a lot of time with the children when they were growing up. Kind and generous to others, except if he thought he was being taken advantage of. When upset often got physically aggressive.
Liked football, walking and other outdoor activities. Loved to work in his allotment.

History
Born in Gateshead. Enjoyed childhood and schooling. Liked his National Service in army. Worked in labouring jobs on the docks and on building sites.
Married at 21 to Sally. Has 3 children and he was a very good father. Sally died 3 years ago.

Environment
In nursing care for the last 2 years.
Socially isolated. Owing to his aggression, attended to in twos by male staff. Staff want him to leave the home.
Regular visits from his sons and daughter. Rarely left his small room. His bed placed at strange angle to wall due to odd shape of room (possible

Mental health
No difficulties between childhood to 65.
Depression after onset of dementia.

Trigger and behaviour
Michael displayed extreme aggression each morning when he saw the male care staff. Tended to attack male carers or females with short hair.

Nature of dementia
Dementia with Lewy body with marked frontal lobe difficulties; resulting in poor attention and disinhibition.
Communication difficulties; prone to misinterpreting situations. Occasionally time-shifted to a time he

Physical health
Bruises down left side of body. Pain; prone to falling. Poor mobility.
Weight loss; very thin/frail.

Need and possible thoughts
The need was revenge! (Safety, self-esteem and having control over his environment.)
Michael believed he was being beaten up by male carers. Hence, he targeted the cares in the morning.

Medication
Memantine, lorazepam.

Vocalisation
When hitting the staff he would say: 'I'll get you ... you bas**rds'; 'I'm not so defenceless now.'

Emotion
Anger.

The items in the grey boxes are the features in the Newcastle Framework that correspond to the CBT cycle (because we usually can't ask about thoughts, we often need to pay attention to what the person is saying in order to get a clue about possible thinking).

Figure 6.3: Simplified version of Newcastle Framework for Michael

The details outlined in Figure 6.3 were agreed in the ISS and were used to develop Michael's care plan. Here are some of the interventions from his care plan:

- Use RAM to identify and gauge his response and the potential risk issues.

- Move the bed further away from the wall to increase his safety and prevent his falls, and install a sensory mat to let staff know when he is getting out of bed.

- To reduce his discomfort, first thing in the morning ask a female staff member to take him a cup of tea and some pain relief.

- Review his medication to see if this may be responsible for falls during night.

- To increase his safety and control over his environment, install a movement sensitive light so a light turns on when he gets up.

- To improve his sense of belonging and relationships, ask the staff to engage more with him during both day and night. Currently the relationship between Michael and staff is very poor; both parties are wary and at times hostile.

As can be seen, several interventions were suggested to deal with the aggression. In this situation many of the strategies were very practical and using this comprehensive approach was helpful to overcome the strained relationship with the staff. The additional information about his history and needs helped his carers to see him as more than just an aggressive man.

TOOLS FOR INFORMING THE FORMULATION AND CARE PLAN

Information regarding occurrence and non-occurrence of behaviours is crucial in understanding their causes and triggers. We can obtain such information through careful observation of the person displaying the behaviour and information from their carers. Here are three types of useful methods and tools:

- *ABC charts.* Useful for observing individual episodes of BtC, and when viewed together, they can help identify behavioural patterns. Such charts are usually called ABC charts because they collect information regarding: the triggers (A – antecedents); the behaviour (B); and the responses to the behaviour (C – consequences). These charts are completed by the carers because they tend to witness the BtC frequently enough to provide information about the patterns to the behaviours.

- *Challenging Behaviour Checklists.* These are lengthy questionnaires in which care staff are asked to identify the type of behaviour, where the BtC took place, potential triggers and potential solutions. The questions are in the form of a checklist, which is designed to be completed in groups, thereby promoting in-group discussion, and can be completed in the presence of clinicians. Although not used routinely, there is an evidence base supporting their use (McCabe, Bird and Davison, 2015; Smith *et al.*, 2016).

- *Normed Scales.* These are frequently used scales, employed to examine the frequency and severity of BtC. Examples include the Challenging Behaviour Scale (Moniz-Cook *et al.*, 2001) or Cohen-Mansfield's Agitation Inventory (Cohen-Mansfield, 1986). They are particularly useful to use before and after an intervention to see if one's therapeutic work has been effective.

Once we have collected information from these tools, we can then put the information together to help decide the likely cause(s). When these details are used in conjunction with the background information from the formulation, we can develop comprehensive care plans.

The best ABC charts should contain enough information to allow any person who was not present during the problematic behaviour to re-enact the event! Unfortunately, ABC charts are frequently done poorly. They often contain too little information and frequently record carers' opinions rather than factual information. For example, one can contrast the difference between 'opinion' and 'fact' in the following accounts of the same incident:

Carer's opinion: Mary got bored with the karaoke and so went to find something more interesting to do.

Factual information: Mary left the room at 12 o'clock, immediately after being asked to sing a karaoke song. She walked into the kitchen and sat down by herself.

The more factual record allows us to speculate about some other reasons, besides boredom, why she left the room, which could include noise or pressure to perform. It therefore helps with the better targeting of our interventions.

CARE PLANS AND TREATMENT SELECTION

Care plans, aka behavioural support plans, are the treatment instructions which have been identified in the formulation. The care plan is the most important document of the whole formulation process, because it specifies the actions that treat the BtC. A care plan should be clear and realistic; the acronym 'SMART' is usually used to describe their features:

S – Specific and clear instructions that provide guidance on what needs to be carried out.

M – Measurable, such that the intervention has a clear start and end.

A – Assigned to an individual or group of people who have responsibility for ensuring the recommendations are carried out.

R – Realistic in terms of the skills and resources available to the staff.

T – Timed in relation to when and where the actions need to be carried out and when a re-evaluation of the interventions' effectiveness is to be conducted.

As we have shown in the case study of Michael, the actions in the care plan are often very practical. To further illustrate this point the box below outlines a summary of the typical sorts of interventions written in care plans from a series of over 100 formulations written by the Newcastle Behaviour Support Team. As you can see, many of the interventions are very practical, although the way they were delivered were different depending on the needs of each PWD.

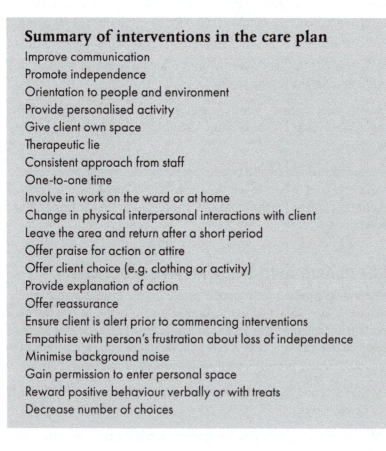

Summary of interventions in the care plan
Improve communication
Promote independence
Orientation to people and environment
Provide personalised activity
Give client own space
Therapeutic lie
Consistent approach from staff
One-to-one time
Involve in work on the ward or at home
Change in physical interpersonal interactions with client
Leave the area and return after a short period
Offer praise for action or attire
Offer client choice (e.g. clothing or activity)
Provide explanation of action
Offer reassurance
Ensure client is alert prior to commencing interventions
Empathise with person's frustration about loss of independence
Minimise background noise
Gain permission to enter personal space
Reward positive behaviour verbally or with treats
Decrease number of choices

An example of a care plan template is provided in Table 6.2.

Table 6.2: Example of a care plan: Smart charts

BtC – identified problem	Treatment	Who assigned to?
Goal of treatment		
Are the interventions SMART (specific, measurable, assigned, realistic, timed)?		
Important things to remember when delivering the intervention with this resident		

THERAPEUTIC LIES

Recent literature has suggested that lying and deception are common within dementia care settings, with 96 per cent of care staff admitting to using lies (James et al., 2006; James and Jackman, 2017). A two year project undertaken by the Mental Health Foundation (2016), in which people with dementia and carers took part, gave cautious support for the use of lies. James et al. (2006) developed guidelines for staff when using lies, to ensure that this form of deception was only employed in line with the best interests of PWD. Research into the reasons for lies/deception being used found common scenarios, such as:

- The PWD believing that a deceased spouse/parent were still alive.

- Easing the distress of PWD who are confused, disorientated and time-shifted.

- Residents and patients wanting to go back to where they previously lived.

In situations such as these, lies are deemed to be acceptable in order to prevent unnecessary distress. Yet they are only considered therapeutic when told for the benefit of the PWD, and they should only be used as the last resort when other approaches have failed (see the Needs Hierarchy, Chapter 4). Below is a framework that is fully consistent with the ethical guidelines.

Guidelines on the use of therapeutic lies

1. Lies should only be told if they are in the best interests of the resident, e.g. to ease distress.

2. Specific areas, such as medication compliance and aggressive behaviour, require individualised policies that are documented in the care plan.

3. A clear definition of what constitutes a lie should be agreed within each setting e.g. the difference between a blatant lie and omission of the truth.

4. Mental capacity assessments should be done on individual patients prior to the use of therapuetic lies.

5. Communication with family members should be required and family consent gained.

6. Once a lie has been agreed it must be used consistently across people and settings.

7. All lies told should be documented.

8. An individualised and flexible approach should be adopted towards each case – the relative costs and benefits established relating to the lie.

9. Staff should feel supported by manager and family; the carer should not feel at risk by telling lies if they have been executed appropriately.

10. Circumstances in which a lie should not be told should be outlined and documented. The relevant circumstances may need to be specified for each resident.

11. The act of telling lies should not lead staff to disrespect the residents – they should be seen as a strategy to enhance the residents' wellbeing, rather than an infringement of their basic rights.

12. Staff should receive training and supervision on the potential problems of lying and taught alternative strategies to use when lies are not appropriate.

This topic remains controversial, but fuller reviews of the concept of the therapeutic lie, and the governance associated with its use, can be found in several recent publications (James and Caiazza, 2018b).

In the final section we explore some of the many non-drug therapies designed to promote wellbeing and reduce BtC. These treatments are often included as part of the PWD's care plans.

NON-DRUG INTERVENTIONS

A major review of non-drug treatments has recently occurred as part of the WHELD trial (Ballard *et al.*, 2018). The trial was a comprehensive examination of treatments and approaches that claimed to enhance wellbeing in people with dementia. Conducted over five years, it examined the evidence-base of treatments and developed some 'best-practice' strategies. It then conducted a controlled-trial examining the benefits of these strategies. Some of the treatments examined in their survey are presented in Table 6.3. The researchers undertook an extensive trawl of studies in the field, looking at the evidence supporting their use. Unfortunately, all of the specific interventions including music, aromatherapy, validation, dance and exercise therapies showed inconsistent findings.

In the final WHELD trial the researchers undertook a major study using the most effective therapies identified. The three interventions used were: (i) social interaction; (ii) person-centred care; and (iii) medication reviews. The results from this study of 60 care homes showed positive results in terms of mortality and BtC.

Table 6.3: Non-pharmacological approaches and their evidence base

Therapies	Systematic reviews and empirical status	Key articles
Reality Orientation: uses rehearsal and physical prompts to improve cognitive functioning related to personal orientation	A Cochrane review by Spector *et al.* (2002) identified six Randomised Controlled Trials (RCTs). The reviewers concluded there was evidence of improvements in terms of cognitive and behavioural features. Reality Orientation is now assessed under Cognitive Stimulation Therapy.	Scanland and Emershaw (1993); Woods *et al.* (2012)
Cognitive Stimulation Therapy: uses structured activities to stimulate mental and physical abilities. Usually undertaken in a structured, group format and derived from RO.	A Cochrane review by Woods *et al.* (2005, updated 2012) suggested that Cognitive Stimulation Therapy had a beneficial effect on memory, cognition and quality of life. Good evidence base for group format, less so for 1:1 packages. Found to be a cost-effective alternative to antipsychotics in reducing distress (NHS III, 2011).	Spector *et al.* (2006); Woods *et al.* (2012); Orrell *et al.* (2014)
Reminiscence Therapy: involves discussion of past experiences individually or in a group format. Photographs, familiar objects or sensory items used to prompt recall and discussion.	A Cochrane review by Woods *et al.* (2005b, updated 2009) identified five RCTs, four containing extractable data. The reviewers reported significant results in terms of cognitions, mood, care-giver strain and functional abilities. However, the quality of the studies was perceived to be poor.	Bohlmeijer *et al.* (2003); Brooker and Duce (2000); Lin *et al.* (2003)
Validation Therapy: based on the general principle of acceptance of the reality of the person and validation of her experience.	A Cochrane review by Neal and Barton Wright (2003, updated 2009) identified three studies, two showing positive effects. However, the reviewers concluded there was insufficient evidence to view the approach as effective.	Schrijne-maekers *et al.* (2002); Feil (1993, 1999)
Psychomotor and Exercise Therapy: exercises (e.g. walking and ball games) are used to target depression and behavioural difficulties. The psychomotor interventions are often targeted at enhancing cognitive abilities in addition to physical wellbeing.	A Cochrane review by Montgomery and Denis (2002) examining the impact of exercise on sleep problems identified one trial that demonstrated significant effects on a range of sleep variables. Teri and colleagues (2008) have undertaken extensive work in this area under the generic title of the Seattle Protocols, and shown evidence of effectiveness for tailored and fun activities.	Eggermont and Scherder 2006; Teri *et al.* (2008)

Multi-Sensory Stimulation: stimuli such as light, sound and tactile sensations, often in specially designed rooms, used to increase the opportunity for communication and improved quality of experience.	A Cochrane review by Chung and Lai (2002, updated 2009) identified a small number of RCTs. A more recent study has shown promising results (Maseda *et al.*, 2014), but was poorly reported. As such, to date there is insufficient evidence to view the approach as effective.	Baker *et al.* (2006); van Weert *et al.* (2005a,b); Maseda *et al.* (2014)
Aromatherapy: use of essential oils to provide sensory experiences and interactions with staff. The oils can be administered via massage techniques or in baths.	A Cochrane review by Holt *et al.* (2009) identified two RCTs, but only Ballard *et al.* (2002) trial reviewed, and found to favour use of essential oils over control oil. More recent trials have mainly failed to find significant effects (AHRQ, 2016).	Ballard *et al.* (2002); Fujii *et al.* (2008); Yang *et al.* (2015)
Bright Light Therapy: use of full spectrum light to enhance wellbeing, increase activity and promote day/night sleeping cycles.	Four good quality trials in area. Reviewed by AHRQ (2016), who concluded that only one trial has shown moderate effects (Burns *et al.*, 2009), and this study has methodological flaws. Forbes *et al.*'s (2014) Cochrane states there is insufficient evidence at this point in time to recommend its use.	Burns *et al.* (2009); Forbes *et al.* (2014)
Music Therapy: includes playing and/or listening to music as a way of generally enhancing wellbeing. Can be used in movement therapies.	A Cochrane review by Vink and Birks (2003, updated 2009) identified five studies. However, the quality of the studies was poor. As such, the reviewers concluded there was insufficient evidence to view the approach as effective.	Sherrat *et al.* (2004); Remington (2002)
Environmental Manipulation: use of environmental cues, signage and appropriate building layout in order to facilitate communication, exercise and pleasure and to reduce disorientation.	The adaption of environments to meet the needs of PWD has been explored extensively by researchers at the DSDC, Stirling University. They have produced a number of successful interventions. Handley *et al.* (2015) have undertaken a review of helpful strategies used in hospital settings to improve outcomes for PWD.	Zuidema *et al.* (2010); Day *et al.* (2000); DSDC (2014)
Behavioural Management Techniques/Functional Analysis: based on learning theory and utilising the antecedents and consequences of behaviour to devise and execute interventions. The approach has a long therapeutic tradition and can be applied to all people, no matter level of cognitive impairment.	A systematic review by Spira and Edelstein (2006) reported 23 studies. These tended to be of poor to moderate quality, and many were single case design. Moniz-Cook *et al.*'s Cochrane (2012) has identified 18 studies with weak but favourable evidence.	Teri *et al.* (2005); Moniz-Cook *et al.* (2012)

From our perspective we believe the findings from WHELD are important because they suggest that the effective non-drug treatments are rather generic in nature. From these results, and the work we have presented in previous chapters of this book, we hypothesise the following:

> Non-pharmacological interventions are effective when they satisfy one or more of people's fundamental needs, and thus they are often multi-sensory. They frequently utilise verbal and non-verbal older memories and can be multi-dimensional. Their success often depends on a person-centred style of delivery, rather than the types or brand of the intervention.

Let us examine the components of the above statement in more detail:

Meeting needs

Effective therapies tend to meet one or more of the eight key needs (Table 2.1). In many respects we should not be asking whether a particular therapy was carried out, rather whether a particular set of needs were fulfilled in accordance with the person's remaining strengths and skills.

Type or brand

There is a wide variety of therapies that have been shown to be effective: aromatherapy, activity/reminiscence box, cognitive stimulation therapy, doll therapy, music, hand massage, reminiscence, simulation presence, animal assisted therapy. However, very few of these types of therapy have shown consistent benefits when assessed in major research trials (NICE, 2018). We hypothesise that in those therapies that have been shown to be effective, the common effective feature has not been the brand of therapy, but rather the manner in which it was delivered because it has satisfied a specific set of needs.

Older memories

Many of the therapies used in dementia care rely on the reactivation of stored memories. These memories can be either verbal or procedural, reminiscence, re-activation of previous skills in hobbies, art, music or activities. An example of a type of procedural (muscle) memory being effective is the HuH™ technique (see Chapters 5 and 7). This approach works because it utilises the long-term neural memories for feeding oneself, cleaning teeth and other self-care activities.

Multi-sensory

Owing to the loss of sensory skills, it is sometimes helpful to present therapeutic materials via several sensory modalities (visual, verbal and tactile). One must be careful, however, not to overload the person's cognitive abilities through over-stimulating them.

Person-centred style vs structure

As Fun Boy Three and Bananarama told us in their song, 'It ain't what you do, but the way that you do it…that's what gets results.' We believe that this statement is true across almost all interventions in dementia care and goes some way to explain why many of our therapies have had such inconsistent outcomes in major research trials.

In the past, too much focus was on the type of intervention, rather than on the process of delivery. We believe the delivery process is often the real intervention and the types of therapies are the vehicles. Hence, a good therapy is simply a vehicle that allows us to meet a range of needs, activates people's memories and is person-centred.

SUMMARY

This chapter has examined the more formal clinical approaches employed by specialist BtC teams. We have examined the problems associated with tranquilising and sedating medications and illustrated alternative approaches which make use of formulations. Some of the charts and questionnaires employed in the area have been mentioned, which can be particularly helpful in identifying the nature of the problematic behaviour and the patterns associated with its occurrence. A list of the non-drug interventions was presented, but concerns were raised because of their lack of a good evidence base.

To account for the lack of consistency of a number of the treatments, we have started to focus on the process of delivery of the treatments rather than brand names. We believe we will have more success in identifying effective change mechanisms if we start to meet people's needs via the methods of delivery of the treatments rather than the type of therapy delivered.

Finally, we suggest that certain types of treatment lend themselves better to meeting people's needs than others, arguing that non-drug interventions tend to be effective when they satisfy one or more of people's fundamental needs, and thus they are often multi-sensory. They frequently utilise verbal and non-verbal older memories and can be multi-dimensional.

References: Chapters 1–6

Agency for Healthcare Research and Quality (AHRQ) (2016) Nonpharmacologic Interventions for Agitation and Aggression in Dementia. Comparative Effectiveness Review Number 177. www.ahrq.gov

Algase, D.L., Beck, C., Kolanowski, A., Whall, A. *et al.* (1996) 'Need-driven dementia compromised behavior: An alternative view of disruptive behavior.' *American Journal of Alzheimer's Disease 11*, 10, 12–19.

Baker, J.C., Hanley, G.P. and Mathews, R.M. (2006) 'Staff administered functional analysis and treatment of aggression by an elder with dementia.' *Journal of Applied Behaviour Analysis 39*, 4, 469–474.

Ballard, C.G., O'Brien, J.T., Reichelt, K. and Perry, E.K. (2002) 'Aromatherapy as a safe and effective treatment fro the management of agitation in severe dementia: The results of a double blind placebo controlled trial with Melissa.' *Journal of Clinical Psychiatry 63*, 553–558.

Ballard, C., Corbett, A., Orrell, M. *et al.* (2018) 'Impact of person-centred care training and person-centred activities on quality of life, agitation, and antipsychotic use in people with dementia living in nursing homes: A cluster-randomised controlled trial.' *PLoS Med 15*, 2, e1002500.

Banerjee, S. (2009) The Use of Antipsychotic Medication for People with Dementia: Time for Action. London: Department of Health.

Banham, M. and Soares, L. (2017) 'When dementia takes leave of our five senses.' *Journal of Dementia Care 25*, 3, 26–29.

Beck, A.T. (1976) *Cognitive Therapy and the Emotional Disorders*. New York: International University Press.

Berne, E. (1964) *Games People Play*. New York: Grove Press.

Bohlmeijer, E., Smit, F. and Cuipers, P. (2003) 'Effects of reminiscence and life review on late-life depression: A metal-analysis.' *International Journal of Geriatric Psychiatry 18*, 1088–1094.

Brooker, D. and Duce, L. (2000) 'Wellbeing and activity in dementia: A comparison of group reminiscence therapy, structured goal-directed group activity and unstructured time.' *Aging and Mental Health 4*, 4, 354–358.

Burns, A., Allen, H., Tomenson, B., Duignan, D. and Byrne, J. (2009) 'Bright light therapy for agitation in dementia: A randomized controlled trial.' *International Psychogeriatrics 21*, 4, 711–721.

Carper, B. (1978) 'Fundamental patterns of knowing in nursing.' *Advances in Nursing Science1*, 1, 13–24.

Chung, J.C.C. and Lai, C.K.Y. (2002, updated 2009) 'Snoezelen for dementia.' *Cochrane Database of Systematic Reviews:* Reviews Issue 4. Chichester: John Wiley & Sons, Ltd.

Cohen-Mansfield, J. (1986) 'Cohen-Mansfield Agitation Inventory (CMAI).' *Journal of the American Geriatrics Society 34*, 722–727.

Cohen-Mansfield, J. (2000) 'Use of patient characteristics to determine non-pharmacological interventions for behavioural and psychological symptoms of dementia.' *International Psychogeriatrics 12*, 1, 373–380.

Day, K., Carreon, D. and Stump, C. (2000) 'Therapeutic design of environments for people with dementia: A review of the empirical research.' *The Gerontologist 40*, 397–416.

DTM Security (2015) The DTM rendition. Dr. George Thompson's '7 things never to say to anyone'. Available at www.youtube.com/watch?v=4BfHPnlnW90, accessed on September 11, 2018.

DSDC (2014) Designing Interiors for People with Dementia. 4th edn. Ed. Liz Fuzzle. Dementia Design Series. Stirling University.

Eggermont, L. and Scherder, E. (2006) 'Physical activity and behaviour in dementia: A review of the literature and implications for psychosocial interventions in primary dementia.' *Dementia 5*, 3, 411–428.

Ellis, M. and Astell, A.J. (2017) *Adaptive Interaction and Dementia: How to Communicate without Speech*. London: Jessica Kingsley Publishers.

Feil, N. (1993) *The Validation Breakthrough: Simple Techniques for Communicating with People with 'Alzheimer's-Type Dementia'*. Baltimore, MD: Health Professions Press.

Feil, N. (1999) 'Current Concepts and Techniques in Validation Methods.' In M. Duffy (ed.), *Handbook of Counselling and Psychotherapy with Older People*. New York: John Wiley.

Flaherty, J.H. (2015) 'Non-pharmacological management of delirium: A proactive approach.' Available at www.americandeliriumsociety.org/blog/non-pharmacological-management-delirium-proactive-approach, accessed on September 11, 2018.

Forbes, D., Blake, C., Thiessen, E., Peacock, S. and Hawranik, P. (2014) 'Light therapy for improving cognition, activities of daily living, sleep, challenging behaviour, and psychiatric disturbances in dementia.' Cochrane Dementia and Cognitive Improvement Group. Available at www.cochranelibrary.com/cdsr/doi/10.1002/14651858.CD003946.pub4/full, accessed on September 11, 2018.

Fujii, M., Hatakeyama, R., Fukuoka, Y., Yamamoto, T. *et al.* (2008) 'Lavender aroma therapy for behavioral and psychological symptoms in dementia patients.' *Geriatrics and Gerontology International 8*, 2, 136–138.

Gibbons, L., Keddie, G. and James, I.A. (2018) 'Investigating the phenomenon of time-shifting.' *Australian Journal of Dementia Care 7*, 1, 32–34.

Glasser, W. (1990) *The Quality School: Managing Students without Coercion*. New York: Harper and Row Publishers, Inc.

Handley, M., Bunn, F. and Goodman, C. (2015) 'Interventions that support the creation of dementia friendly environments in health care: Protocol for a realist review.' *Systematic Reviews 4*, 180.

Hamdy, R. , Lewis, J., Copeland, R., Depelteau, A. Kinser, A., Kendall-Wilson, T. and Whalen, K. (2018a) 'Repetitive questioning exasperates care-givers.' *Gerontology and Geriatric Medicine 4*.

Hamdy, R., Kinser, A., Depelteau, A., Lewis, J., Copeland, R., Kendall-Wilson, T. and Whalen, K. (2018b) 'Repetitive questioning II.' *Gerontology and Geriatric Medicine 4*.

Hamdy, R., Kinser, A., Kendall-Wilson, T. *et al.* (2018c) 'Impulsive, disinhibited behavior: Dining in a restaurant.' *Gerontology and Geriatric Medicine*, Mar 14, 4, 2333721418756994.

Health Education England (2018) Dementia Training Standard Framework. Available at www.hee.nhs.uk/our-work/dementia-awareness/core-skills, accessed on October 05, 2018.

Holle, D., Halek, M., Holle, B. and Pinkert, C. (2016) 'Individualized formulation-led interventions for analyzing and managing challenging behavior of people with dementia – an integrative review.' *Aging and Mental Health 21*, 12, 1247–1249.

Holt, F.E., Birks, T.P.H., Thorgrimsen, L., Spector, A., Wiles, A. and Orrell, M. (2009) 'Aroma therapy for dementia.' *Cochrane Database of Systematic Reviews 4*, 4, CD003150.

Houston (2015) 'Dementia and Sensory Challenges – Dementia can be more than memory.' Booklet and DVD, Life Changes Trust. Available at www.lifechangestrust.org.uk/news/dementia-and-sensory-challenges-booklet-published, accessed on September 12, 2018.

James, I.A. (1999) 'Using a cognitive rationale to conceptualise anxiety in people with dementia.' *Behavioural and Cognitive Psychotherapy 27*, 4, 345–351.

James, I.A. (2010) *Cognitive Behaviour Therapy with Older People: Interventions for Those with and without Dementia.* London: Jessica Kingsley Publishers.

James, I.A. (2011) *Understanding Behaviour in Dementia that Challenges.* London: Jessica Kingsley Publishers.

James, I.A. (2015) 'The use of CBT in dementia care: A rationale for Communication and Interaction Therapy (CAIT) and therapeutic lies.' *The Cognitive Behaviour Therapist 8,* e10.

James, I.A. (2018) 'Therapeutic lies.' Keynote Presentation at Behaviour and Cognitive Therapy Conference. Strathclyde University. July.

James, I.A. and Jackman, L. (2017) *Understanding Behaviour in Dementia that Challenges.* 2nd edn. London: Jessica Kingsley Publishers.

James, I.A. and Caiazza, R. (2018a) 'Transactional Analysis in dementia care.' *Psychology of Older People: The FPOP Bulletin.* BPS, 141.

James, I.A. and Caiazza, R. (2018b) 'Therapeutic lies in dementia care: Should psychologists teach others to be person-centred liars in dementia care?' *Behavioural and Cognitive Psychotherapy 46*, 4, 454–462.

James, I.A., Carlson-Mitchell, P., Ellingford, J. and Mackenzie, L. (2007) 'Promoting attitude change: Staff training programme on continence care.' *PSIGE Newsletter 97*, 11–16.

James, I.A. and Hope, A. (2013) 'Relevance of emotions and beliefs in the treatment of behaviors that challenge in dementia patients.' *Future Medicine 3*, 6, 575–588.

James, I.A. and Moniz-Cook, E. (2018) Evidence briefing: behaviour that challenges in dementia. British Psychological Society. www.bps.org.uk

James, I.A., Wood-Mitchell, A., Waterworth, A.M., Mackenzie, L. and Cunningham, J. (2006) 'Lying to people with dementia: Developing ethical guidelines for care settings.' *International Journal of Geriatric Psychiatry 21*, 800–801.

Kitwood, T. (1997) *Dementia Reconsidered: The Person Comes First.* Buckingham: Open University Press.

Lin, Y.C., Dai, Y.T. and Hwang S.L. (2003) 'The effect of reminiscence on the elderly population: A systematic review.' *Public Health Nursing 20*, 4, 297–306.

Macaulay, S. (2015) 'B is for breathe in BANGS: Care partnering, challenging and solutions, tips and tools and skills.' *My Alzheimer's Story,* June 18. Available at www.myalzheimersstory.com/2015/06/18/b-is-for-breathe-in-bangs, accessed on September 12, 2018.

Mackenzie, L. and James, I. (2010) 'How a time machine concept aids dementia care.' Available from ianandrew.james@ntw.nhs.uk.

Mackenzie L., Smith, K. and James, I. (2015) 'How a time machine concept aids dementia care.' *Nursing Times, 111*, 17, 18–19.

Maseda, A., Sánchez, A., Marante, M.P., González-Abraldes, I., Buján, A. and Millán-Calenti, J.C. (2014) 'Effects of multisensory stimulation in a sample of institutionalized elderly people with dementia diagnosis: A controlled longitudinal trial.' *American Journal of Alzheimers Disease and Other Dementias 29*, 463–473.

Maslow, A.H. (1943) 'A theory of human motivation.' *Psychological Review 50*, 4, 370.

Maslow, A.H. (1954) *Motivation and Personality.* New York: Harper and Row.

McCabe, M.P., Bird, M. and Davison, T.E. (2015) 'An RCT to evaluate the utility of a clinical protocol for staff in the management of behavioral and psychological symptoms of dementia in residential aged-care settings.' *Aging & Mental Health 19*, 9, 799–807.

Mehrabian, A. (1972) *Non-verbal Communication.* Chicago, IL: Aldine-Atherton.

Mehrabian, A. (1981) *Silent Messages: Implicit Communication of Emotions and Attitudes.* 2nd edn. Belmont, CA: Wadsworth.

Mental Health Foundation (2016) 'What is truth? An inquiry about truth and lying in dementia care.' London: MHF.

Moniz-Cook, E., Woods, R., Gardiner, E., Silver, M. and Agar, S. (2001) 'The Challenging Behaviour Scale (CBS): Development of a scale for staff caring for older people in residential and nursing homes.' *British Journal of Clinical Psychology 40*, 309–322.

Moniz-Cook, E., Walker, A., De Vugt, M., Verhey, F. and James, I. (2012) 'Functional analysis based interventions for challenging behaviour in dementia (Cochrane Review).' *Cochrane Database of Systematic Reviews.*

Montgomery, P and Dennis, J. (2002) 'Physical exercise for sleep problems in adults aged 60+.' *Cochrane Database of Systematic Reviews 4.* Chichester: John Wiley & Sons, Ltd.

Neal, M. and Barton Wright, P. (2003, updated 2009) 'Validation therapy for dementia.' *Cochrane Database of Systematic Reviews 3.* Chichester: John Wiley & Sons, Ltd.

NICE (2018) 'Dementia: Assessment, management and support for people living with dementia and their carers.' Guidance/ng97.

NHS Institute for Innovation and Improvement (2011) An economic evaluation of alternatives to antipsychotic drugs for individuals living with dementia is published by the NHS Institute for Innovation and Improvement, Coventry House, University of Warwick Campus, Coventry, CV4 7AL.

O'Connor, E., Caiazza, R. and James, I. (2017) 'A response framework with untruths as last resort.' *The Journal of Dementia Care 25*, 4, 22–25.

Orrell, M., Aguirre, E., Spector, A., Hoare, Z. *et al.* (2014) 'Maintenance Cognitive Stimulation Therapy (CST) for dementia: A single-blind, multi-centre, randomised controlled trial of Maintenance CST vs. CST for dementia.' *British Journal of Psychiatry 6*, 454–461.

Patterson, S.M., Hughes, C., Kerse, N. *et al.* (2012) 'Interventions to improve the appropriate use of polypharmacy for older people.' *The Cochrane Database of Systematic Reviews 16*, 5, CD008165.

Pool, J. (2012) The Pool Activity Level (PAL) *Instrument for Occupational Profiling: A Practical Resource for Carers of People with Cognitive Impairment.* 4th edn. London: Jessica Kingsley Publishers.

Ranka, J. and Chapparo, C. (1997) 'Definition of Terms.' In C. Chapparo and J. Ranka (eds), *Occupational Performance Model (Australia): Monograph 1* (pp.58–60). Sydney: Occupational Performance Network.

Remington, R. (2002) 'Calming music and hand massage with agitated elderly.' *Nursing Research 51*, 5, 317–323.

Royal College of Psychiatrists (2011) Report of the National Audit of Dementia Care in General Hospitals 2011. London: Healthcare Quality Improvement Partnership.

Schrijnemaekers, V., Vanrossum, E., Candel, M. *et al.* (2002) 'Effects of emotion oriented care on elderly people with cognitive impairment and behavioural problems.' *International Journal of Geriatric Psychiatry 17,* 926–937.

Scanland, S.G. and Emershaw, L.E. (1993) 'Reality orientation and validation therapy. Dementia, depression, and functional status.' *Journal of Gerontological Nursing 19*, 6, 7–11.

Sherratt, K., Thornton, A. and Hatton, C. (2004) 'Music interventions for people with dementia: A review of the literature.' *Aging and Mental Health 8,* 3–12.

Smith, K., Hadaway, L., Reichelt, K. and James, I. (2016) 'The Newcastle Challenging Behaviour Checklist: Feedback about its use in the treatment of agitation.' *FPOP Bulletin 134,* British Psychological Society.

Snow, T. (2012) *Dementia Care-giver Guide: Teepa Snow's Positive Approach Techniques for Care-giving, Alzheimer's and Other Forms of Dementia.* Mason, OH: Cedar Village.

Sorokowska, A., Sorokowski, P., Hilpert, P. *et al.* (2017) 'Preferred interpersonal distances: A global comparison.' *Journal of Cross-Cultural Psychology 48*, 4, 577–592.

Spector, A., Orrell, M., Davies, S. and Woods, R.T. (2002) 'Reality orientation for dementia (Cochrane review).' In *The Cochrane Library.* Update Software, issue 2: Oxford.

Spector, A., Thorgrimsen, L., Woods, B. and Orrell, M. (2006) *Making a Difference: An Evidence-Based Group Programme to Offer Cognitive Stimulation Therapy (CST) to People with Dementia.* London: Hawker Publications.

Spira, A. and Edelstein, B. (2006) 'Behavioral interventions for agitation in older adults with dementia: An evaluative review.' *International Psychogeriatrics 18*, 2, 195–225.

Stokes, G. (2006) 'Responding to the Need to Toilet.' In G. Stokes and F. Goudie (eds), *The Essential Dementia Care Handbook*. Bicester: Speechmark Editions.

Tanner, L. (2017) *Embracing Touch in Dementia Care: A Person-Centred Approach to Touch and Relationships*. London: Jessica Kingsley Publishers.

Teri, L., Logsdon, R.G. and McCurry, S.M. (2008) 'Exercise interventions for dementia and cognitive impairment: The Seattle Protocols.' *The Journal of Nutrition, Health and Aging 12*, 6, 391–394.

Teri, L., McCurry, S.M., Logsdon, R. and Gibbons, L.E. (2005) 'Training community consultants to help family members improve dementia care: A randomized controlled trial.' *The Gerontologist 45*, 6, 802–811.

Thompson, G. and Jenkins. J. (2013) *Verbal Judo: The Gentle Art of Persuasion*. New York: HarperCollins Press.

Van Weert, J.C., Van Dulmen, A.M., Spreeuwenberg, P.M., Ribbe, M.W. and Bensing, J.M. (2005a) 'Behavioral and mood effects of snoezelen integrated into 24-hour dementia care.' *Journal of the American Geriatrics Society, ISSN (PRINT VERSION): 0002 8614,* 53, 24–33.

Van Weert, J.C., Van Dulmen, A.M., Spreeuwenberg, P.M., Ribbe, M.W. and Bensing, J.M. (2005b) 'Effects of snoezelen, integrated in 24 h dementia care, on nurse–patient communication during morning care.' *Patient Education and Counseling ISSN (PRINT VERSION): 0738 3991,* 58, 312–326.

Vink, A.C. and Birks, J.S. (2003, updated 2009) 'Music therapy for people with dementia.' *The Cochrane Database Reviews*. The Cochrane Database of Systematic Reviews.

Wilcock, A. (1993) 'A theory of the human need for occupation.' *Journal of Occupational Science 1*, 1, 17–24.

Woods, B., Spector, A.E., Prendergast, L. and Orrell, M. (2005, updated 2012) 'Cognitive stimulation to improve cognitive functioning in people with dementia.' *Cochrane Database of Systematic Reviews: Protocols Issue 4.*

Woods, B., Spector, A., Jones, C., Orrell, M. and Davies, S. (2005b, updated 2009) 'Reminiscence therapy for dementia.' Cochrane Database of Systematic Reviews: Reviews Issue 2.

Yang, M-H., Lin L-C, Wu, S-C., Chiu, J-H., Wang, P-N. and Linm, J.G. (2015) 'Comparison of the efficacy of aroma-acupressure and aromatherapy for the treatment of dementia-associated agitation.' *Bio Med Central Complementary and Alternative Medicine 15*, 93.

Zuidema, S., de Jonghe, J., Verhey, F. and Koopmans, R. (2010) 'Environmental correlates of neuropsychiatric symptoms in nursing home patients with dementia.' *International Journal of Geriatric Psychiatry 25*, 1, 14–22.

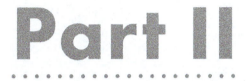

Part II

Chapter Seven

Enhancing Care-Givers' Communication Skills

Teepa Snow's Positive Approach to Care™ (PAC™) and GEMS™

SUSANNAH THWAITES

This chapter outlines the main concepts of Positive Approach to Care™ (PAC™) and describes how this approach has been used within Tees, Esk and Wear Valleys NHS Foundation Trust (TEWV) to develop communication skills in care-givers. The latter is illustrated using case studies.

OVERVIEW OF POSITIVE APPROACH TO CARE™

Teepa Snow, a dementia specialist in the USA, developed Positive Approach to Care™ (Snow, 2012) to support people living with dementia by equipping both formal and informal carers with specific skills and to increase their understanding of what it is like to live with dementia. Her approach is focused on interactions and care delivery. Two concepts that are central to the use of PAC™ are GEMS™ and the Positive Physical Approach™ (PPA™). GEMS™ is a six-item rating system based on the Allen Cognitive Levels (Allen, 1982), which highlights the strengths of people with dementia (PWD) and guides the nature of interactions required from care-givers to meet PWD's needs. The Positive Physical Approach™ describes practical steps for engaging and interacting with PWD, taking account of cognitive, sensory and emotional changes.

GEMS™

The GEMS™ concept helps others to see people living with dementia as precious gems (Sapphire, Diamond, Emerald, Amber, Ruby and Pearl). The focus is on what skills remain, rather than what is lost; in PAC™ it is the preferred alternative to PAL (Chapter 5). The GEMS™ explains the changes in the brain and why people living with dementia may behave in a certain way (Table 7.1). It supports the care partner to be flexible in his approach and helps to make care partnering easier by matching the carer's approach with the specific needs of the individual. Teepa Snow suggests that in the right setting, with the right care, all GEMS™ can shine (Snow, 2012). This fits well with what Tom Kitwood (1990) described as being central to person-centred dementia care, namely that the environment and the response and interactions of carers are crucial to the person being able to experience wellbeing.

Table 7.1: The GEMS™ framework with features
and skills associated with each gem

Sapphire Normal ageing with a healthy brain	True to self: personal preferences remain basically the same
	Can be flexible in thinking and appreciate multiple perspectives
	Stress/pain/fatigue may trigger Diamond state: back to Sapphire with relief
	Able to suppress and filter personal reactions: chooses effective responses
	Selects from options and can make informed decisions
	Processes well and able to successfully transition
	Ageing doesn't change ability: processing slows, more effort/time/practice needed
Diamond Clear and sharp with routines ruling	Displays many facets: behaviour and perspective can shift dramatically
	Prefers the familiar and may resist change
	More rigid and self-focused; sees wants as needs when stressed
	Personal likes/dislikes in relationships/space/belongings etc. become more intense
	Reacts to changes in environment; benefits from familiar
	Needs repetition and time to absorb new/different information or routines
	Trusted authority figures can help: reacts better when respect is mutual
Emerald Green and on the go with a purpose	Sees self as able and independent, with limited awareness of changes in ability
	Can be 'time-shifted': awareness of time, place and situation will not always match current reality
	Understanding and use of language change: vague words and many repeats
	Cued by what they see
	Strong emotional reactions are triggered by fears, desires or unmet needs
	Needs to know what comes next: seeks guidance and assistance to fill the day

Amber Caught in a moment of time, caution required	Focused on sensation: seeks to satisfy desires and tries to avoid what is disliked
	Environment can drive actions and reactions without awareness of safety
	Visual abilities are limited: focus is on pieces or parts, not the whole picture
	What happens to or around an Amber may cause strong and surprising reactions
	Enters others' space and crosses boundaries attempting to meet own needs
	Has periods of intense activity: may be very curious or repetitive with objects or actions
	Care is refused or seen as threatening, due to differences in perspective and ability
Ruby All fine motor skills stop but strength remains	Makes use of rhythm: can usually sing, hum, pray, sway, rock, clap and dance
	When moving can't stop; when stopped can't get moving: needs guidance and help
	Big, strong movements are possible, while skilled abilities are being lost
	Danger exists due to limited abilities combined with automatic actions or reactions
	Tends to miss subtle hints, but gets magnified facial expressions and voice rhythms
	Can mimic actions or motions, but will struggle to understand instructions/gestures
	Able to pick up and hold objects, and yet does not know what to do with them
Pearl Hidden within a shell, beautiful moments to behold	Will frequently recognise familiar touches, voices, faces, aromas and tastes
	Personhood survives, although all other capabilities are minimal
	Understanding input takes time: go slow and simplify for success
	In care, first get connected by offering comfort then use careful and caring touch
	Changes in the body are profound: weight loss, immobility, systems are failing
	As protective reflexes are lost, breathing, swallowing and moving will be difficult
	Care partners benefit from learning the art of letting go rather than simply giving up

The GEMS™ concept encourages care partners to assess 'in the moment' which GEM™ the person 'is' and respond with the appropriate cues to support them. It acknowledges that PWD's skills and abilities fluctuate across a day, depending if they are unwell or if they are anxious or distressed. Indeed, many of us without dementia may start off the day as a flexible and quick-thinking Sapphire, but at the end of a stressful day will be intolerant of others, will only be able to do things the way we always do them and have difficulty with solving complex problems, in other words, we become a Diamond. A PWD may start off the day as an Emerald and by teatime, due to, for example, fatigue, sensory overload or experiencing pain, may be presenting as an Amber. The care partner needs to recognise this, be flexible and adapt their approach accordingly.

Positive Physical Approach™ and Hand under Hand™

Another key concept to PAC™ is Positive Physical Approach™, including Hand under Hand™ (HuH™), which is a practical method of working with the PWD to connect and deliver care on a variety of levels. These techniques have already been described and referred to in Chapters 4 and 5.

A central principle in PPA™ is to connect with the person first using visual cues, then verbal cues and finally touch cues. If we touch a PWD without first giving a visual and a verbal cue, we are more likely to elicit a negative response and may trigger a behaviour that challenges (BtC). According to PPA™, the type of touch that we should use during many personal care interventions is a light, moving touch. This is detected by the tactile receptors in our skin and is transmitted along nerve pathways to stimulate the amygdala, sometimes referred to as the emotional centre of the brain. During many tasks, we are also focusing on areas of the body that have the highest concentration of tactile receptors, such as the genitals or mouth area. These areas are naturally more sensitive.

A person who is still able to reason with the frontal lobe of their brain will know that they are being helped and be able to tell themselves: 'They are nurses and they are helping me, it's okay.' However, if that part of the brain is damaged and frontal function is impaired, the person may react instinctively to what the brain is telling them and perceives this interaction as a threat or danger (Ayres, 2005). The steps of PPA™ and some of the rationale are outlined in the box below; note the similarities to what was described in Chapter 4.

Positive Physical Approach™

Approach the person from the front – so if they have a limited visual field they can see you coming

Pause at 6 feet – get permission to enter their personal space

Give 'Hi' sign and say 'Hi!' – give a visual and a verbal cue

Use their name and tell them your name – make a personal connection

Offer a handshake – this is a visual cue that says 'I want to come into your personal space and I want to touch you'

Go slow – reaction times get slower as we age

Move from a handshake to the Hand under Hand™ position

Get to the side of the person – be supportive, not confrontational

Get low – do not use your height to intimidate; kneel or sit

Be friendly – say something nice, greet and compliment, introduce yourself again

The Hand under Hand™ technique can be used in a variety of ways; to provide connection, to gain and maintain attention, to provide substitution for skilled activities and tool use, to redirect unwanted touch and to provide reassurance.

Pressure in the palm of the hand, especially at the base of the thumb, is calming and relaxing to the nervous system. It stimulates the release of the neurotransmitter oxytocin (Ziesel, 2009), which leads to feelings of caring and reassurance, and decreased stress and anxiety. It does the opposite to the alerting light touch.

As people progress through dementia, they will lose skill, but keep strength. For example, Ambers will start off by being able to use a fork or spoon, but as they lose more skill they may need finger foods to remain independent. Rubies lose fine motor skills so have difficulty using cutlery or holding a toothbrush but can still grip tightly and carry things.

Care partners can use HuH™ to support PWD by becoming the skill for the person, whilst giving a sense of control and involvement; doing *with* not *to* the person. HuH™ uses eye-hand coordination, which is one of the first sensorymotor loops developed when we are infants. It is used as we learn to do tasks that become stored in our motor memory, which are then automatic to us. By using HuH™, using motor memories and creating a closed circuit in the brain, we are less likely to alert the fight or flight system. This is what happens when we touch ourselves – we know what is coming and we are not startled by it.

Connecting with the different GEM™ states

In our experience, there are common challenges that arise with each GEM™ state. We have outlined some tips to help care partners respond in a positive way (Table 7.2). Some of the advice is consistent with other techniques described in Chapter 4, such as DATA and BANGS, but this section is more centred on the person's current skills and abilities.

Table 7.2: Connecting with the GEM™ states

Connecting with Diamonds	• Do not argue with the person – this will only cause confrontation
	• Give up reality orientation – this will only highlight their deficits to them and cause more arguments
	• The 'I'm sorry's' can be really useful:
	  – 'I'm sorry I made you…angry/sad/frustrated/anxious/feel stupid'
	  – 'I'm sorry this happened'
	  – 'I'm sorry, this is hard'
	  – 'I'm sorry, you're right' – be willing to give up being right
	• If the person asks or tells you something repeatedly, don't say 'Remember I already told you.' Instead try to:
	  – repeat the gist of what the person said
	  – offer the information they asked about
	  – keep your voice calm and friendly
	  – respond and then get the person onto another subject by asking for their help with something
	• Don't come across as bossy or trying to take over. Stop saying 'I can't let you do…', instead ask them to help you, or say 'Can we try this?' Avoid making the person feel incompetent or highlighting that they are unable to do something

Connecting with Emeralds
 	
Emeralds may be time-shifted, especially as the day goes on and they will ask to go places or see people that are from their past.
	• Go with the flow and don't challenge the person's reality – try to figure out where they are at that point in time. If the person asks to go home or says they are looking for their mother, be careful not to argue or use reality orientation:
	  – First repeat the person's words – don't answer the question – 'You need to get home,' 'You are feeling a need for your mother'
	  – Then make an emotionally supportive comment such as 'You've always loved being at home…', 'Sounds like you are really missing your mother…' – make sure you pause and listen to what they say
	  – If the person can converse say 'Tell me about your home/your mother'
	  – If language is a problem, offer information about the person or the place such as 'You have something you need to do at home…?' or 'Is your mother a great cook? Do you like dinners or puddings better?' – this is not distraction, but redirection
	• Greet before you treat – it is important to establish the relationship rather than going straight in and trying to address something that you noticed is wrong or needs fixing. If you want the person to do something, use a visual cue first; show the person by pointing, gesturing, use a prop or demonstrate or do it alongside them, not to them
	• The art of substitution (of the behaviour) not subtraction – ask the person if they can help you rather than pointing out that they need the help or need to stop doing something
	• If they have word finding problems useful phrases are: 'Tell me more about it', 'Show me what you do with it.' Offer the person 'either/or' choices, e.g. 'Would you like tea or coffee to drink?', rather than 'What do you want to drink?'

Connecting with Ambers	• It is important to realise their understanding is limited and that they will not benefit from explanations or reassurance, especially when anxious/distressed • They will still be able to get the rhythm of speech and so will get a lot of meaning from the paraverbals – the way we say things • We need to keep verbal instructions to a couple of words (less is more) and match with a gesture or non-verbal cue • If they are being supported with care tasks, make sure only one person does the talking if there is more than one carer needed – agree beforehand who is going to lead • The HuH™ approach can be used to guide and assist when helping the person, rather than doing it for them
Connecting with Rubies	• Comprehension and speech production will be very limited • They may have some social chit chat. They will still have the rhythm of speech but it will be difficult to make sense of • Can often still sing so we can use music and rhythm to connect, initiate movement, slow down or liven up. We need to know their personally meaningful music • Demonstrate and show the person what you want them to do, rather than telling them or getting louder • If you want the person to slow down or do something, start where they are and then gradually change the speed or rhythm with your pace and voice. Use what is calming to the person to help settle them and what is stimulating to them to get them going again • Use HuH™ guidance for assisting with movement and point with your other hand where you want them to go or what you want them to notice. Also use HuH™ to provide touch or care as it gives the person more information that makes sense to their brain and limits the over-sensitivity in the very sensitive areas of the body, where care is often needed
Connecting with Pearls	• Reflexes rule the body and care is focused on providing comfort and moments of connection with the person • Connect with comforting sensory-based experiences. Consider use of Namaste care (Simard, 2013) • Go slow, be calm – the person needs lots of time to process things • Use your tone of voice to convey reassurance • We need to stay in touch – keep one hand on the person's shoulder, hip, hand or back with an open palm to steady and stabilise, and use the palm of the other to give care

Our team have used the guidance above from PAC™, combined with information from Psychological Formulation, Nursing or Occupational Therapy Assessment to develop more detailed, individualised interventions and Behaviour Support Plans and shared these with our care partners. In TEWV, we are rolling out PAC™ training within in-patient teams, community teams, delivering training to care home staff and are beginning to share these ideas with family carers. It is then an opportunity for training to be further embedded and put into action when an individual we are working with has a Behaviour Support Plan developed that incorporates PAC™.

CASE STUDIES

The following are Behaviour Support Plans that have been developed either collaboratively with care home staff and family at a formulation meeting or following an Occupational Therapy assessment. These examples demonstrate how PAC™ has enabled some detailed interventions to be generated. Most of the examples relate to Stop Start Scenarios (SSS) (James and Hope, 2013), as discussed in Chapter 4. PAC™ often is part of the primary preventative or sometimes secondary reactive strategies. The focus is to reduce the likelihood that distress and BtC occur.

Case study: Chris is functioning as a Diamond, who needs to feel in control

BEHAVIOUR SUPPORT PLAN

Patient Name: Chris   **DoB:** 1950   **Date:** June 2017

Description of the behaviour(s) that challenge

- Chris shouts and swears at care staff when he does not gain their support straight away and he will demand to speak to the manager.

What are the person's needs that may be causing this behaviour?

- Chris has changes in the frontal lobe of his brain, which means he has difficulty with supressing impulses to say/do rude or inappropriate things (but can still remmber doing them and may even be sorry about them), is not able to see other people's points of view and is impatient. This means he comes across as demanding and selfish.

- Chris is frustrated as he needs support from staff due to his limited mobility. He needs to feel like he is in control of some aspects of his life as he used to have a job where he was in a position of authority and was used to being in charge of people.

Aims

- Staff to be aware of how Chris's brain change is impacting on his behaviour and functioning.
- Staff to respond to Chris in a way that does not cause a confrontation.

Things that we do all the time to improve Chris' quality of life and reduce the likelihood of behaviours that challenge

- Avoid telling him what to do/what not to do.
- Instead give him choice over every little thing you ask him to do to increase his feeling of control e.g. 'Do you want to come to the dining room now or wait a while?', 'Do you want to wear this or that?', 'Would you like a cold drink or hot one?'
- Also ask his advice on things – tell him how smart he is and that you value his input.

Things that cause/trigger the behaviours to occur

- When Chris makes a request of staff that cannot be immediately responded to.
- Staff trying to explain to him that they are busy and there are others who need their help more than he does.
- Telling him he will have to wait.
- If he feels he is being told what to do.

How Chris may appear just before and during the behaviour that challenges

- Chris raises his voice, tells staff they are useless and should be sacked and that he wants to see the manager about them.

Things to do when we notice a behaviour occurring or getting worse

- Don't criticise Chris or tell him what he has done is 'inappropriate' – reflect that you can tell he is angry and apologise/tell him he is right
- 'I'm sorry's' – such as 'I'm sorry I made you angry', 'I'm sorry you're right, I shouldn't have done that', 'I'm sorry you've had to wait, you're right it's not good enough, I apologise' etc.

Case study: John is functioning at Emerald level as the day progresses and becomes time-shifted

BEHAVIOUR SUPPORT PLAN

Patient Name: John   **DoB:** 1943   **Date:** April 2018

Description of the behaviour(s) that challenge

- John is becoming agitated from 4pm to around 8.45pm. He shouts at staff, bangs on the lift doors and can then hit staff.

What are the person's needs that may be causing this behaviour?

- John is time-shifted and often thinks he is in his old workplace at the university. He is cued by teatime that he should be getting himself home and leaving for the day, and so when prevented from doing so becomes increasingly distressed as he thinks he is being held against his will.

Aims

- To increase staff skills in responding to John's distress when he thinks he needs to leave.

Things that we do all the time to improve John's quality of life and reduce the likelihood of behaviours that challenge

- As teatime approaches, try supporting John to have his tea in his bedroom to make him feel like he has left for the day to go to his own place. We know that he used to like watching the news and quiz programmes around this time of day so make sure the TV is on the appropriate channel.

Things that cause/trigger the behaviours to occur

- Teatime, which is the time when he should be getting himself home after work and leaving for the day. This is also a busy and noisy time of day on the unit with lots of comings and goings.

How John may appear just before and during the behaviour that challenges

- A sign that John is about to become distressed is when he says 'What are you looking at?'

- He will ask to leave saying 'What authority do you have to keep me here?' and then shout that the police need to be called and say that staff cannot keep him here.

- He often focuses on the lift area as he knows it is the way out.

Things to do when we notice a behaviour occurring or getting worse

- When John is time-shifted and thinks he should be going home at the end of the 'working' day:

  – Keep tone of voice calm but it may help to mirror John's expression as this will help him to know you understand what he is trying to tell you

  – Be careful not to argue or use reality orientation – go with the flow

  – First repeat the John's words – don't answer the question – 'You need to get home'

  – Then make an emotionally supportive comment such as 'You've always been on time for tea' – make sure you pause and listen to what he says

  – Engage him in conversation related – say 'Tell me about your home/your family', 'Who's the cook in your house?' – this is not distraction but redirection

  – Redirect him to a new activity and a new place by asking for his help with something.

Case study: Marion is an Amber who is exploring her environment

BEHAVIOUR SUPPORT PLAN

Patient Name: Marion   **DoB:** 1948   **Date:** February 2018

Description of the behaviour(s) that challenge

- Marion goes into other resident's bedrooms and picks up and takes objects that she finds. Marion becomes angry with staff and can try to push them.

What are the person's needs that may be causing this behaviour?

- Marion is not orientated around the unit and is not aware that some areas are other people's private space which leads to her going into other's bedrooms.

- She is a lady who liked to be busy and she has a need for sensory input, as she likes the feel of 'and to fiddle with' the things she finds.

- When staff try to get her to leave or try to take an object off her she can interpret this as a confrontational situation and become angry.

Aims

- To increase staff's skills in redirecting Marion when she is in others' rooms.

- To provide opportunities for Marion to explore, feel busy and gain the sensory tactile input she is seeking.

Things that we do all the time to improve Marion's quality of life and reduce the likelihood of behaviours that challenge

- Marion needs objects to search out and engage with. Place rummage boxes with a variety of interesting things she can feel and fiddle with around the unit. Leave some out in plain view and others under chairs or slightly out of the way so she can explore.

- When Marion is in someone else's bedroom, staff should not criticise Marion or say 'no' – she has no awareness that she is in someone else's space and could easily interpret trying to redirect her as a confrontation.

- Greet Marion by saying her name in a friendly way and offer a handshake and then move into the Hand under Hand™ position.

- Remark that she looks busy and offer to help her.

- Offer Marion a cup of tea and biscuit, gesture drinking and say 'Come with me, let's have a break, we'll put the kettle on.'

- Alternatively ask for her help with something. If she needs a stronger, visual cue, have a basket of things that need folding with lots of colour and different textures. We know she was very house-proud and liked to help others.

- Then make sure you support her to engage in either of the above in a different part of the building.

Things that cause/trigger the behaviours to occur

- When she feels like staff are stopping her from doing what she feels she needs to do.
- When she is guided out of the bedroom and told she can't be in there.
- When objects are taken out of her hands.

How Marion may appear just before and during the behaviour that challenges

- Marion says 'it's mine' when they try to take things from her.
- When staff try to guide her out of the room she sometimes looks angry and pushes them.

Things to do when we notice a behaviour occurring or getting worse

- First ask if you really need to remove the object from Marion's possession right now – can it wait until she puts it down?
- Try offering her a swap for a chocolate biscuit or another object such as the bright sparkly cushions which we know are very attractive to her.

Case study: Rose functions as a Ruby when being supported with personal care

BEHAVIOUR SUPPORT PLAN

Patient Name: Rose   **DoB:** 1936   **Date:** June 2018

Description of the behaviour(s) that challenge:

- Rose is physically aggressive when being supported to change following incontinence. She will bite, kick, grab and hit staff.
- She also hits staff at other times and staff say there is 'no trigger' at these times.

What are the person's needs that may be causing this behaviour?

- The type of touch used during personal care is known to alert the fight or flight part of the brain which can take over if someone cannot think things through and control their impulses effectively. Rose reacts instinctively to protect herself from what she perceives as a threat as she thinks staff are trying to touch her private parts inappropriately. She cannot understand the situation or benefit from explanations for reassurance due to her communication difficulties.

- Rose may hit out at other times due to the changes in her visual field and being startled when approached.

Aims

- To reduce distress during personal care interventions.

Things that we do all the time to improve Rose's quality of life and reduce the likelihood of behaviours that challenge

- Approach Rose from the front getting her attention with a visual cue and offer a handshake which tells her, without words, that you intend to enter her personal space and touch her.

- Move from the handshake into a Hand under Hand™ position and also move to the side, and if she is seated get down to her level.

Things that cause/trigger the behaviours to occur

- Being supported following an episode of faecal incontinence.

- People getting in her personal space and coming from the side.

How Rose may appear just before and during the behaviour that challenges

- Rose bites, kicks, grabs and hits out at staff when they are supporting her. She screams and shouts 'No, get off.'

Things to do when we notice a behaviour occurring or getting worse

- Approach Rose using the above technique to connect with Hand under Hand™.

- Rose needs two carers to support her with personal care but one carer needs to lead and give her slow and gentle instructions in the form of gestures as to what is happening to her and the other carer needs to keep 'quiet'.

- Using Hand under Hand™ may help to reduce triggering/alerting Rose's flight or fight response by using deep pressure type touch which is more calming to the nervous system. By supporting her own hand during the interaction, it will trick her brain into thinking she is doing the activity herself and it will feel less invasive.

Case study: Andrew is a Pearl in need of connection

BEHAVIOUR SUPPORT PLAN

Patient Name: Andrew   **DoB:** 1939   **Date:** April 2017

Description of the behaviour(s) that challenge

- Screaming, nipping and scratching staff.

What are the person's needs that may be causing this behaviour?

- Andrew is sensitive to noise and needs calm and quiet. He was observed to startle, and then shout out, about the noise when a cupboard door near his bedroom was shut.

- He has difficulty filtering environmental information and becomes easily over stimulated by noise.

Aims

- To engage Andrew at the 'just right' level to match his cognitive abilities.

- To reduce sensory overload.

Things that we do all the time to improve Andrew's quality of life and reduce the likelihood of behaviours that challenge

- Andrew may benefit from having short periods in the quieter communal areas interspersed with periods in his bedroom.

This will minimise sensory overload due to noise but allow him to have a change of scene/environment.

- When engaging with Andrew remember to go slow and use your voice to convey reassurance as he needs lots of time to process things. Connect with HuH™ if this is comfortable for him.

- Continue to use music for short periods across the day either in his bedroom or if he spends time in the quieter lounges. This will be most effective if it is music that is to his personal taste so use of the radio should not be encouraged.

- Develop a Namaste care box to provide gentle and relaxing sensory experiences tailored to the individual so that staff and family can spend time at regular intervals engaging with Andrew. Contents could include:

  - Elvis Presley and Buddy Holly CDs
  - Small bag of compost to smell as he was a keen gardener
  - Bottle of 'Old Spice' aftershave, which was his favourite when going 'out on the town' as a young man
  - Soft blanket he can be wrapped in as he used to always complain of the cold
  - Olive oil so that gentle hand massage can be used.

Things that cause/trigger the behaviours to occur

- Being in the bigger communal lounge due to noise.
- Having too many people in his room.

How Andrew may appear just before and during the behaviour that challenges

- Andrew screams loudly and will reach out and nip or scratch staff's arms when they approach him.

Things to do when we notice a behaviour occurring or getting worse

- If Andrew starts to shout or scream support him to access a quieter space.
- Try putting on some of his favourite music.
- Make sure he has one of his soft blankets on.

Implementation of PAC™

In Tees, Esk and Wear Valleys NHS Foundation Trust, two occupational therapists trained as PAC™ Trainers when Teepa Snow came to the UK for the first time in 2015. Since then a further six occupational therapists have undertaken the training. The occupational therapists in Older People Services within TEWV have been using the Allen Cognitive Levels (Allen, 1982) for many years, so were in a good position to lead the development of PAC™ within the Trust, as Teepa Snow's GEMS™ framework is based on the Allen model. The Pool Activity Level (PAL) discussed in Chapter 5 was also derived from the Allen model, but we have found the GEMS™ to be more meaningful and memorable for staff and carers. In TEWV Trust, PAC™ training has been undertaken with approximately 500 care home staff. CAIT has been delivered alongside this by a clinical psychologist, to complement the PAC™ training (James, Marshall and Thwaites, 2017).

SUMMARY

This chapter has outlined how Teepa Snow's Positive Approach to Care™ and the GEMS™ model has been used to support care-givers in implementing individualised interventions that match with the person's current cognitive abilities. To conclude here are some PAC™ general rules for connecting with all PWD:

- Use visual, verbal and then touch cues in that order, but be mindful of adapting PPA™ for each GEMS™ state.

- Be in the moment – ask yourself 'Where is the person right now?'

- Gauge their emotion and mirror it, coming in just below where they are – show the person you understand what they are trying to communicate.

- Make a personal connection before you try to do some activity with the person – it's your relationship that is important, not what you want to get done.

- Be aware that the PWD will take more notice of our appearance and behaviour rather than the words we use, and so facial expression and gestures are important.

- Do things *with* the PWD not *to* them.

REFERENCES

Allen, C.K. (1982) 'Independence through activity: The practice of occupational therapy (psychiatry).' *American Journal of Occupational Therapy 36*, 11, 731–739.

Ayres, A.J. (2005) *Sensory Integration and the Child*. 2nd edn. Los Angeles, CA: Western Psychological Services.

James, I.A. and Hope, A. (2013) 'Relevance of emotions and beliefs in the treatment of behaviors that challenge in dementia patients.' *Future Medicine 3*, 6, 575–588.

James, I., Marshall, J. and Thwaites, S. (2017) 'Improving communication skills in dementia care: Utilising the British Psychological Society's stepped-care model for treatment of behaviour that challenges.' *FPOP Newsletter 137*, 36–41.

Kitwood, T. (1990) 'The dialectics of dementia: With particular reference to Alzheimer's disease.' *Aging and Society 9*, 1–15.

Simard, J. (2013) *The End-of-Life Namaste Care Program for People with Dementia*. 2nd edn. Baltimore, MD: Health Professions Press.

Snow, T. (2012) *Dementia Care-giver Guide: Teepa Snow's Positive Approach Techniques for Care-giving, Alzheimer's and Other Forms of Dementia*. Mason, OH: Cedar Village.

Ziesel, J. (2009) *I'm Still Here*. New York: Penguin Group.

Chapter Eight

Promoting Consent to Touch During Personal Care

LUKE TANNER

INTRODUCTION

This chapter examines the topic of consent to touch during care tasks that require care-givers to have some form of physical contact with people with dementia (PWD). Consent, which is also often referred to as 'permission giving', is essential in order that the recipient of the touch does not feel violated, attacked or used. I discuss the topic from a practical and informal perspective, and do not examine the legal and governance issues associated with the topic, which have been discussed elsewhere (Sells and Howarth, 2014). However, before examining the issue of consent in detail, it is worth highlighting the breadth and dynamic nature of human contact. Figure 8.1 presents a summary of my typology of touch (Tanner, 2017). This typology of touch can help us to understand the role different kinds of touch play in shaping personhood, relationships and wellbeing.

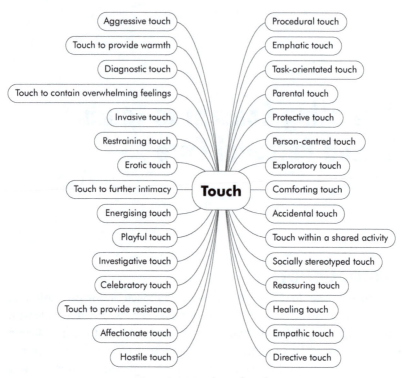

Figure 8.1: Typology of touch

CONSENT TO TOUCH

Many of the tasks required to support PWD necessitate some physical contact. This means that PWD, particularly those living within residential care settings, are often being touched during personal care tasks over the course of a day. Having a cognitive impairment can have a profound impact on how someone experiences being touched because many PWD neither have insight into their care needs nor understand a carer's intentions or verbal explanations when receiving help. Furthermore, because some people's verbal language skills reduce over the course of a dementia, they will increasingly rely more on their experience of touch to make sense of the situation and relationship with others.

This shift from verbal to tactile communication can therefore totally transform experiences of touch in care tasks from something reasonable and desirable to something extremely stressful, hostile and even traumatic. In some cases, PWD can respond by engaging in distressed behaviours such as kicking, screaming, swearing or scratching. These responses can have a devastating effect on carers and PWD alike.

For carers, such behaviours can lead to high stress, physical injury and even burn-out. For PWD, we may see the emergence of stigmatisation or isolation, as well as the development of serious health problems including malnutrition, dehydration and infection owing to care-giver avoidance. The behaviours can also function to break the bridge of trust and affection so vital for the giving and receiving of care.

The problematic behavioural responses to touch during care tasks have often been misperceived as symptoms of dementia and referred to variously as resistance to care and non-compliant and aggressive behaviour. Unfortunately, these terms do not help us to understand the underlying cause of these behaviours nor help us to alleviate them. Labelling PWD as resistant, non-compliant or aggressive and framing the latter behaviours as a symptom of dementia implies that either the person or their dementia is the cause of the problem.

Recognising such behaviours as behavioural responses to touch invites us to reflect on the implications of our use of touch in the care of PWD. Furthermore, identifying the factors that determine our experiences of touch can help us discover ways of promoting consent to care tasks without having to rely upon someone's logic and reasoning.

Experiences of touch cannot simply be determined by the type of touch (i.e. area of contact, pressure, duration), because the experiences change across situations, within different relationships and are dependent upon the nature of the body language. These factors are all crucial to our experience of touch and whether someone consents to touch or not. Four key factors that help us to examine the overall experience of the physical contact are presented below.

- *The type of touch* – how someone is touched. This includes the quality of touch, what part of the body is touched, the duration of the touch and whether the touch is given and/or received.

- *The situation* – why, where and when the touch occurs. This aspect includes the context in which the touch occurs: timing, intention and environment.

- *The relationship* – who is touching whom. This factor refers to the attributes of the individuals who are in touch, such as familiarity, personality, life experience, gender, social role, culture, religion, identity.

- *Body language* – what people do when they are touching. This feature refers to posture, proximity, facial expression, eye contact and breathing.

Carers of PWD can work creatively with the four factors to obtain consent on those occasions when someone is initially reluctant to engage in the care activity. With knowledge of the factors to consent, carers can do far more than merely achieve consent and can turn care tasks into meaningful relationships and emotionally fulfilling activities. This can alter PWD's lived experience of care and enhance their quality of life.

DISTINGUISHING PERSON-CENTRED FROM TASK-ORIENTATED TOUCH
Person-centred

Person-centred touch is about *being* with someone and is reciprocal. Much of the touching that occurs in everyday life relates to our identity and emotional needs. These forms of touch are such an everyday aspect of social life that it is easy to forget the crucial role they play in shaping who we are and how we feel. A handshake can meet our need for identity; sitting close beside someone can meet someone's need for inclusion; holding someone's hand can meet someone's need for comfort; a hug can meet someone's need to feel safe and secure (attachment).

Task-oriented

In contrast, task-oriented touch is about *doing* something and tends to be one way, i.e. the person doing the task is the one doing the touching and the touch is about addressing someone's physical needs. This form of touch is goal-oriented as it focuses on the completion of a given task. A person may feel some comfort and relief after the task is complete, but it is not the actual experience of touch that is comforting or reassuring.

Whilst touch is a pervasive feature of dementia care, what types of touch occur in each care setting has a lot to do with the wider culture of care. Given that the quality of touch in care determines the quality of caregiving relationships, a carer's approach to touch will always be a key determinant of the lived experience of care. In the next section we will examine the potential impact of task orientated environments on people's illbeing.

TASK-ORIENTED CULTURES OF CARE

In care settings where people's physical needs have come to take precedence over people's emotional needs, touch will become confined to care tasks and procedures. In these clinical care settings such tasks and procedures will be scheduled at particular times of the day and organised into rigid caregiving routines. Examples of people's experience of touch in care are outlined in the box below.

People's experiences of being touched

grasped	gripped	shuffled	stood up
held	fastened	nudged	sat down
lifted	pushed	caught	brushed
dropped	pulled	released	rubbed
positioned	leaned	squeezed	wiped
secured	carried	swiveled	hoisted

Being constantly touched in this way is likely to make someone feel more like an object rather than a person worth meeting. Such experiences can result in people feeling disempowered and controlled and can have a huge impact on a person's experience of relationships. After all, how human beings are touched inevitably shapes how they feel about themselves and their relationships with others. This is particularly the case with PWD who rely more on their experience of touch to make sense of their relationships due to their cognitive impairment. Seen in this context it might seem more understandable why some people might respond to being touched in care tasks with behaviours of protest or withdrawal.

Care-resistant behaviours can tell us something about the wider culture of care and staff's use of touch. In many task-oriented cultures of care, in which routine-bound care rules the day, PWD may be handled as if they were an object or moved as if they were a piece of furniture as a matter of routine. In this context someone's care-resistant behaviours should be recognised as a sign of illbeing.

RESISTANCE TO TASK-ORIENTED TOUCH

Task-oriented touch involves some loss of control over some of the factors crucial to our experience of touch. This loss of control means that touch tends to trigger the very states we spend most of our lives avoiding, such as: anxiety, stress, fear, shame, vulnerability, confusion. These feelings can be triggered by all sorts of events, from a dental check-up to an invasive surgical procedure. We consent to these forms of touch not because the touch itself is satisfying but because we are confident that the outcome of the task is desirable. We consider the consequences of not having the doctor's examination, dental procedure or medical treatment and recognise the potential for more severe discomfort or greater distress. In short, we recognise that the 'end justifies the means'.

Our capacity to rationalise the experience not only makes it reasonable, but more bearable. Unfortunately, many PWD cannot rely on this logical reasoning since dementia can undermine this capacity. Many PWD cannot recognise that in some cases their experience of touch is a function of a given care task. This turns an examination, procedure or treatment into an experience of a very hostile, invasive, aggressive or even abusive relationship. The kicking, screaming or shouting are therefore very natural responses to this experience of touch. It is very difficult to suppress, inhibit or bring these behaviours under conscious control during states of extreme stress and even more so when experiencing severe cognitive impairment.

Within dementia care these fight or flight behaviours are often labelled as 'resistance to care'. Seen from the perspective of someone who cannot rely on logic and reason to make sense of the task, these tasks are anything but caring.

EXAMPLES OF PROMOTING CONSENT TO TOUCH IN PERSONAL CARE

Many carers rely on people's logic and reasoning to promote consent when people are resistant to care, but they are appealing to the very capacity that has been impaired. In the examples that follow carers develop extraordinary approaches that do not rely on logic or reasoning and which achieve highly positive results.

Case study: Elizabeth

Elizabeth was in an advanced stage of dementia and living in a residential dementia care home. Elizabeth did not have sufficient insight into her need to wash and could neither make sense of the process involved in getting into the bath nor why someone needed to assist her in this activity. Lacking this awareness, Elizabeth was resistant to any carer's attempts to wash and clean her. Staff attempts to attend to this basic need often led to Elizabeth shouting, kicking, scratching and even biting the carers involved.

Elizabeth had developed a reputation in the home as being aggressive and some staff became very wary of her, avoiding contact with her both within and outside care tasks. Elizabeth's personal hygiene seriously deteriorated as a result. Her anti-social behaviour and poor personal hygiene resulted in increasing isolation and stigmatisation. However, one carer had noticed that Elizabeth enjoyed humming religious hymns and discovered that one of her favourite hymns was 'Onward Christian Soldiers'.

Elizabeth liked to keep busy around the home by participating in household and caregiving activities. The staff at the home always ensured that they had some items around for Elizabeth to pick up and use to occupy herself, such as carpet sweepers, tea towels, cleaning cloths, a pram and some baby dolls.

The carer decided to draw on this knowledge of Elizabeth in her approach to washing and bathing her. She began by sitting down and spending some time with her while Elizabeth cared for her dolls. They began to bathe the dolls and sing 'Onward Christian Soldiers' together. Through these activities Elizabeth was able to see what washing and bath time involved, that is was safe and that the carer's involvement was worthwhile. Since discovering this approach carers have managed to help her bath without upset or resistance. In fact, Elizabeth now thoroughly enjoys her bath time.

To promote consent to this care task, staff began by spending time with Elizabeth to develop a *relationship* characterised by trust and affection. They adapted their *body language* to convey this kind of relationship, beginning the task by sitting down. This kind of body language expresses a willingness to *be with* Elizabeth rather than *do something to* her. They then used dolls and singing to adapt the caregiving *situation* in which the use of *touch* was two-way so that it met Elizabeth's need to care and nurture someone. Elizabeth had an opportunity to touch and bathe the doll before being touched and bathed herself. While meeting Elizabeth's need for good personal hygiene, this enriched care task also met her need for meaningful occupation and belonging.

Case study: Iris

Iris was a Londoner living in a residential care home in Nottingham. She was experiencing a different reality as a result of her level of cognitive impairment; she was often worried about her husband, who had already passed away, and getting her daughters to school, who had long grown up. Iris needed assistance with personal care and was often reluctant to receive this help. One afternoon Iris had soiled herself and needed personal care, but any carer who tried to do anything about it was met with rebukes and offensive remarks, 'F**k off'; 'You need to clean *yourself* up you dirty b**tard!' However, no matter how discreet, kind and polite the carers were in their approach, Iris responded in the same manner, hitting out if carers got too close. Different carers tried but to no avail. One carer felt that maybe Iris needed somebody else, somebody she could relate to, so she left the room and changed her clothing and hair. She put on a denim jacket, let down her hair and put on a bowler hat. She returned in this new attire and this time talked in a cockney accent. She made a point of referring to her colleagues as the dirty, silly b**tards and suggested she get rid of the lot of them so the two of them could sort things out. Iris decided to go with the cockney person who appeared to be on her side, rather than the other carers who were 'just being a pain in the a**e'.

To promote consent to this intimate care task the carer had to become someone else. Iris could relate to another cockney woman, who talked like her. This turned out to be the *relationship* that Iris felt safest in at her time of need. To develop this relationship, the carer had to get into role, changing her language, accent, *body language* and clothing.

METHOD IN THE MADNESS

An analysis of the above examples demonstrates that consent to a given care task depends on one or more of the following factors: *the type of touch, the situation, the relationship and body language*. In the examples given above carers worked with one or more of these factors to develop caregiving relationships and situations that secured consent (see Figure 8.2).

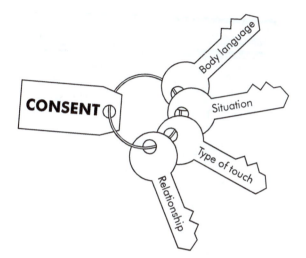

Figure 8.2: Keys to consent

The first step to achieving consent is to recognise that we are not doing a care task to someone but in fact creating a relationship with someone. Taking this step essentially means letting go of the targeted task. In the examples given above the carer lets go of the task to form a relationship with the other person. Since the quality of the relationship is so fundamental to our experience of touch, developing a relationship characterised by trust, familiarity and affection can be enough to promote consent. A heightened awareness of non-verbal communication is an important part of this relationship-centred approach to consent. When words mean less, the messages we convey with our body will mean a lot more. A carer can demonstrate this awareness by doing something very simple, like sitting down! Sitting and standing postures can convey very powerful messages. While sitting down conveys the messages, 'I am here to be with you' and 'It's safe here'; standing up can mean, 'I have something to do' and 'I am on the move.'

Promoting consent can also mean not just letting go of the set task for a moment or two: it may involve re-inventing the task altogether, working with the *situation*. This proved to be the case with Elizabeth. Bathing Elizabeth became Elizabeth bathing a baby. Instead of trying to make these activities reasonable, the carer simply made them more emotionally fulfilling. With sufficient motivation, people who lack mental capacity can be encouraged to engage with an activity without the insight or understanding ordinarily required for verbal consent. Motivating someone who lacks capacity to understand a given care task means making that task meet an emotional need alongside the physical care need (see Figure 8.3).

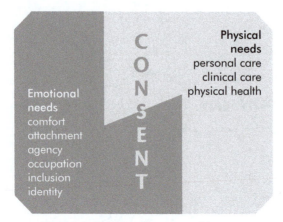

Figure 8.3: Conditions for non-cognitive consent

In this case someone is motivated to do something based on how they *feel* rather than what they *think*. This kind of consent could be called 'non-cognitive consent'. While verbal consent relies on a given task being a reasonable thing to do, 'non-cognitive consent' relies on the task itself *feeling* like a good thing to do. That means that every care task needs to be emotionally appealing. Since this relies on a more instinctive response, these activities needed to be shaped by the recipient's changing feelings and needs. Hence, the caregiving situations described above were improvised. Like in childhood play, carers needed to make up the rules and change roles as they go along, surprising themselves with how things unfold. Carers approached these personal care tasks more like games to play than jobs to get done.

NON-COGNITIVE CONSENT AND A PLAYFUL CULTURE OF CARE

Promoting non-cognitive consent can look a lot more like playing and hanging-out than 'working' and getting things done. In professional care settings, this playful approach involves making dynamic risk assessments in order to obtain non-cognitive consent. Such risk assessments may at times involve transgressing some of the standard care practices. Carers can struggle to achieve this form of consent if they feel fearful of breaching such standards and norms.

Professional care organisations can promote the above approach by recognising the capacity of their employees to make dynamic risk assessments that lead to creative personal care interventions. Therefore organisations need to grant greater freedom to their care staff, and also give them sufficient time to play. This means relaxing caregiving routines and going with the flow.

Finally carers also need to be given the means to play. Elizabeth and Iris's carers worked in caregiving environments filled with stuff for them to draw on and experiment with. This enriched caregiving environment is absolutely essential to experimentation and play. In contrast, in clinical environments that are impersonal and empty it is extremely difficult to transform a situation into something more meaningful. Enriching a dementia care environment with a variety of novelty items, comfort objects, sensory items and things that relate individual life history enables the carers to adapt a caregiving situation to someone's unique needs with greater ease.

SUMMARY

Consensual caregiving depends on a sufficient degree of both trust and motivation. This is the case with every recipient of care. How a carer develops that trust and motivation, however, differs from one person to the next. A carer must therefore have a sense of the individual they are caring for and an insight into the things that really matter to them to achieve consent. This means reflecting on the characteristics and qualities of the people that the individual tends to trust and the kind of activities that were a source of meaning to them in the past. With this informed and intuitive approach, carers can develop the trusting relationships and meaningful caregiving situations that promote real consent to care.

Just as a person with dementia needs to trust in their carers enough to consent to care, care providers need to trust in their staff enough for them to create unconventional approaches to conventional care tasks. The professional carers involved in the examples above trusted in themselves, their colleagues and their managers. They all worked within a culture of care in which experimentation, spontaneity and thinking outside the box were considered part and parcel of dementia care. This approach to consent is only possible within a culture of care that gives carers the freedom to:

- let go of the task at hand
- do things differently
- follow their insights and intuition
- be creative and spontaneous
- draw on comfort objects, novelty items and things relating to individual life history
- adapt care practices to unique human needs.

A care provider's capacity to reduce care-resistant behaviours will be largely determined by the extent to which its culture of care trusts its staff and grants them this freedom.

REFERENCES AND FURTHER READING

Dean, R., Proudfoot, R. and Lindesay, J. (1993) 'The Quality of Interactions Schedule (QUIS): development, reliability and use in the evaluation of two domus units.' *International Journal of Geriatric Psychiatry 8*, 10, 819–826.

Fleischer, S., Berg, A., Zimmermann, M., Wüste, K. and Behrens, J. (2009) 'Nurse–patient interaction and communication: A systematic literature review.' *Journal of Public Health 17*, 5, 339–353.

Fredriksson, L. (1999) 'Modes of relating in a caring conversation: A research synthesis on presence, touch and listening.' *Journal of Advanced Nursing 30*, 5, 1167–1176.

Gilbert, D. (1998) 'Relational message themes in nurses' listening behavior during brief patient-nurse interactions.' *Scholarly Inquiry for Nursing Practice: An International Journal 12*, 1, 5–27.

Gleeson, M. and Timmins, F. (2004) 'Touch: A fundamental aspect of communication with older people experiencing dementia.' *Nursing Older People 16*, 2, 18–21.

Kitwood, T. (1997) *Dementia Reconsidered: The Person Comes First.* Buckingham: Open University Press.

Knocker, S. (2015) *Loving: The Essence of Being a Butterfly in Dementia Care.* London: Hawker Publications Ltd.

Le May, A.C. and Redfern, S.J. (1987) 'A Study of Non-Verbal Communication between Nurses and Elderly Patients.' In P. Fielding (ed.), *Research in the Nursing Care of Elderly People.* London: John Wiley & Sons, Ltd.

Le May, A.C. and Redfern, S.J. (1989) 'Touch and Elderly People.' In J.W. Wilson-Barnett and S. Robinson (eds), *Directions in Nursing Research: Ten Years of Progress at London University.* London: Scutari Press.

Montagu, A. (1986) *Touching: The Human Significance of the Skin.* New York: William Morrow Paperbacks.

Routasalo, P. (1996) 'Non-necessary touch in the nursing care of elderly people.' *Advanced Nursing, 23*, 5, 904–911.

Routasalo, P. (1999) 'Physical touch in nursing studies: A literature review.' *Advanced Nursing, 30*, 4, 843–850.

Routasalo, P. and Isola, A. (1996) 'The right to touch and be touched.' *Nursing Ethics 3*, 2, 165–176.

Sells, D, and Howarth, A. (2014) 'The Forced Care Framework: Guidance for staff.' *Journal of Dementia Care 22*, 6, 30–34.

Sheard, D.M. (2014) 'Achieving culture change: A whole organisation approach.' *Nursing and Residential Care 16*, 6, 329–332.

Tanner, L. (2014) 'Reaching towards deeper levels of communication.' *Journal of Dementia Care, 22*, 1, 26–28.

Tanner, L. (2017) *Embracing Touch in Dementia Care: A Person-Centred Approach to Touch and Relationships in Care.* London. Jessica Kingsley Publishers.

Ward, R., Vass, A.A., Aggarwal, N., Garfield, C. and Cybyk, B. (2008) 'A different story: Exploring patterns of communication in residential dementia care.' *Ageing & Society 28*, 5, 629–651.

Chapter Nine

Adaptive Interaction

Facilitating Communication in Advanced Dementia

MAGGIE ELLIS AND ARLENE ASTELL

BACKGROUND

When dementia reaches very advanced stages, those living with a diagnosis typically inhabit a socially impoverished environment. Changes in the communicative abilities of individuals with dementia eventually reach a stage at which producing speech is no longer possible. As such, communication *as we recognise it* becomes impossible. At this very late stage, the person with dementia may also have lost his ability to walk or to engage in any personal care activity without assistance. As such, he is likely to spend the majority of his time in bed, completely dependent on the care of others. As he *appears* to have lost his ability to communicate, professional care-givers and family members make fewer attempts to interact with him over time and the person with dementia becomes an observer rather than a participant in the social world. This situation plays out time and time again in care facilities across the world and it is untenable.

The following chapter offers an alternative to the preceding scenario. In it we discuss a communication intervention called Adaptive Interaction (AI) and a trainee's experiences of learning how to use and engage in the technique in everyday care. Our research shows that despite the loss of ability in terms of producing speech, people with advanced dementia retain the *desire* to communicate with others. Perhaps more surprisingly, we have shown that individuals with advanced dementia also retain the *ability* to interact. However, the loss of spoken language means that communication skills in people with advanced dementia appear very different to our everyday interactions. As such, in order to engage in this form of interaction, we must first change our minds about what it means to communicate. This is no small feat considering we have spent a lifetime using speech to communicate with others. It is undoubtedly challenging to reconsider the purpose and forms of communication, but it is both possible and necessary if we are to engage with individuals with advanced dementia. In order to change minds, we must change practice and as such, this chapter also explores the barriers to using AI in the care environment and how we can overcome these.

ADAPTIVE INTERACTION

Adaptive Interaction (Ellis and Astell, 2017a) is a non-verbal communication technique that requires users to reconsider what it means to communicate and to engage with an alternative realm of interaction. AI was developed specifically for individuals with advanced dementia and is a variant of Intensive Interaction (II) (Hewett, 1996; Nind, 1996). Intensive Interaction or II was established in the 1980s as a method of communicating with individuals with profound and multiple learning disabilities and reflects the principles of how infants develop the ability to interact with others.

We are born with a set of communicative behaviours known as the 'fundamentals of communication', which include actions such as touch, movements and sounds. In healthy babies, these very basic actions develop over time in conjunction with the engagement of our parents and other adults and we very quickly learn that our actions have an impact on other people and the world around us. The following is an example of such an interaction taken from our book on Adaptive Interaction (Ellis and Astell, 2017b, p.55).

> Imagine…that you are visiting a friend who has a two-month-old baby. After a short while, your friend asks you if you wouldn't mind looking after the baby for 20 minutes while he pops out to the shop. You have never had a baby of your own and are more than a little apprehensive about what 'to do' with her. However, you agree to look after her while your friend runs an errand. The moment your friend leaves the house, you start to feel self-conscious and doubtful as to your ability to care for the infant. However, she is asleep and you sit down to wait for your friend to return. Then you hear a sound from the crib and realise the baby is waking up. She makes a sound and you get a little closer to see what she is doing. The baby immediately spots you and you smile at her – quite instinctively. She responds to you with a smile. You smile again and she keeps looking at you and smiling. Then you repeat the sound she made and she keeps her eyes on yours. Then you try another sound and she keeps looking and

she makes a sound. Then you smile again and the two of you are having a 'conversation'. However, you don't feel that you need to speak to the baby. Nevertheless, what you both understand from this exchange is that you are interested in each other, are happy to be together and have, in some way, connected. The communication that you have engaged in with the baby is more about 'feeling' something than conveying a message. You have communicated without words on perhaps a deeper level than you might if you could talk to each other.

There are two key elements to this interaction. First is the importance of *reflecting* or imitating what we hear, see and feel in others, which is absolutely essential to the development of communication skills. Second is *behaviour matching* in the other direction, as parents naturally imitate the actions of their babies, effectively letting the infant know that she is being attended to. Via this collaboration with others, our communication skills develop quickly to include facial expressions, direction of eye gaze, turn-taking and eventually speech.

Those of us who develop atypically (e.g. individuals born with learning disabilities, congenital deaf-blindness or autistic spectrum disorder) may never learn to speak or to understand speech. However, we know that these individuals develop their own repertoires of the fundamentals of communication, e.g. sounds, movements, facial expressions, etc. (Caldwell and Horwood, 2007). As with young infants, we do not assume that these alternative interactions are non-communicative. Rather, we are likely to work with the communicative repertoires displayed by these individuals. In other words, we engage with their own individual 'language' (Caldwell, 2007).

Intensive Interaction makes use of the communicative repertoires of individuals who have developed atypically to engage with them, to develop relationships and to involve them in learning activities over time (Nind, 1996; Hewett, 1996). The approach has a growing evidence base and is recognised by a number of key professional bodies as a valid method of engaging with people who have developed atypically. Intensive Interaction affords the atypically developed person entry into a social world that would be unavailable to them via traditional communication methods, i.e. speech. Excited by this approach, we recognised the potential of II to possibly reengage people with advanced dementia with the social world and we were eager to pursue this line of research. However, we were also very aware of the possible challenges of teaching professional carers how to engage in this approach and of gaining the acceptance of the academic community.

We first attempted to apply the principles of II to engage with a single person with advanced dementia named Edie. Edie was an 80-year-old woman who had been resident in a care home for six years when we first met her. She was no longer able to walk or to take care of other personal needs without assistance. By this stage of her illness, Edie was also no longer able to speak and to the untrained eye appeared to be completely non-communicative. However, our observation over two days in her care environment revealed that Edie *did* make attempts to engage with others but that these were not recognised as such by staff members and were largely ignored. For example, Edie made a very loud signature sound that staff and residents found to be disturbing and as a consequence, she was confined to her bedroom for most of the day. We found that by reflecting instead of ignoring this sound we afforded Edie the opportunity to engage with another person using elements of her *own* language (Ellis and Astell, 2017b). She engaged with the researcher (communication partner) using turn-taking, sounds, movements, facial expressions, touch and – perhaps most surprisingly – smiling and laughter (Ellis and Astell, 2008).

One important aspect of II is that once a connection is made between a non-verbal individual and an interaction partner, this is built on over time to develop a communication model for each individual (Caldwell, 2008). However, dementia is a progressive neurological disorder whereby people experience longitudinal impairment in memory and other cognitive processes. If they reach the point of being non-verbal, they will have experienced pronounced changes in memory and other aspects of cognition. As such we could not presume that we could involve individuals with advanced dementia in learning activities as achieved in II to build up their communication skills. Rather, we decided to focus on simply connecting with the person in the moment and adapting to whatever they are doing at any given point. This approach requires the communication partner to meet the person where they are and to adapt their interaction accordingly. As such, we named this variant of II 'Adaptive Interaction'.

This early success encouraged us to conduct further research in this area and we have now engaged with scores of individuals with advanced dementia using AI. Our research shows that AI provides the means for people with advanced dementia to demonstrate their retained abilities and unique communication repertoires comprising a variety of non-verbal components, spanning eye gaze, emotion expression, sounds and movement (Ellis and Astell, 2017b). These findings confirm the potential of Adaptive Interaction as the basis for interacting with people living with dementia who can no longer speak.

We have also developed a tried and tested AI training programme to help staff and family members engage with individuals with advanced dementia. For the purposes of this chapter we return to the beginning of this part of the AI story, to the very first AI training we conducted. We have refined and formalised the training programme considerably since this first attempt; however, we feel that this early example will provide the reader with an honest example of the aforementioned challenges faced by both trainees and trainers.

TRAINING PROGRAMME

Three employees (a nurse, an activities coordinator and a care assistant) of a local care home agreed to take part in the AI training. Four training sessions of two hours each were delivered over a five-week period. The training programme was developed by the authors using an active learner model, providing theoretical background information and incorporating practical activities for trainees to practise between sessions. The approach also encouraged the staff participants to share their experiences and support each other in the use of AI.

The first session consisted of providing a brief introduction to the training and pairing trainees with people with advanced dementia. The first author (M.E.) then explained the theoretical background and aims of AI. Finally the staff were provided with a video camera and asked to make a five minute video of a 'typical' interaction between themselves and the resident with whom they had been paired. The second and third training sessions adopted a very similar format. Within these sessions, the trainees made video recordings of themselves with their communication partners, now engaging in AI. In each session staff were given sheets listing seven fundamentals of communication: sounds, eye gaze, facial expression, physical contact, vocalisations, gestures and turn-taking. They were then asked to complete the sheets, indicating if any of the fundamentals occurred, while they watched the videos of their own interactions with the people with dementia they were working with. Additionally, during both sessions, the staff were shown videos of the author (M.E.) interacting with a person with dementia using verbal communication and using AI. During the third training session the staff were also given a handout describing communication skills in healthy infants, severe autism and people with dementia.

During the final training session the staff also assessed their own videos for the fundamentals of communication. Furthermore, as this was the last training session, the focus was placed on how they could take the technique further and continue to apply it during their everyday practice. The staff were also given a handout with a more detailed explanation about the theory supporting AI. A follow-up session took place two weeks after the end of the training to gain feedback about the course from the staff and a final session took place two weeks after the follow-up session and included family members of participants with advanced dementia and the care-givers who took part in the training. During the session M.E. explained the findings of the study and showed video clips of AI being used to facilitate interactions between the care staff and people with advanced dementia.

FINDINGS

The findings of the AI training programme revealed three main points. First, trainees were enabled to identify the fundamentals of communication in people with advanced dementia. This meant that trainees were able to recognise communicative behaviours as deliberate attempts to engage rather than viewing them as meaningless and random. Second, trainees thought that the people with dementia with whom they communicated throughout the programme had improved in terms of their interactions. This, of course, is unlikely in view of the progressive nature of dementia. What is more likely to have happened here is that staff became more aware of communicative actions and that this therefore changed how they viewed the person with dementia. Third, the findings showed that it is possible to train care and nursing staff in the principles of AI and that through this they gain new knowledge and skills that can improve the lives of individuals with advanced dementia. These main findings were crucial to the further development of AI as an intervention and to the training programme itself.

The trainees were interviewed six months after the training in order to assess their feelings about both the training and AI itself. These interviews were also integral to how AI is now framed by us when we teach care staff and nursing staff in how to use the approach, and just as importantly, how to continue using it. The following is a transcript from an interview with one of the trainees – a nurse. It illuminates the obstacles that she experienced in trying to keep going with AI after the training, and she also suggests how the approach could be implemented more widely in the care environment.

Trainee 1: Nurse

M.E. (author): Please talk to me about the main things you have learned during the training.

Nurse: The main things I learned were that non-verbal communication is far more beneficial to a lot of our clients than trying to communicate verbally because a lot of them are further on in their dementia. Also, instead of trying to communicate with someone at the other end of the room – being in their space, being in front of them, eye contact and at their level.

M.E.: Do you think the training made a difference to how you do your job?

Nurse: 'Yeah – with certain clients, yeah. It makes you think a bit more when you're communicating. Like when you're trying to get something across. For example, sometimes you're trying to communicate verbally then all of a sudden you remember the training course. Sometimes a particular resident gets very agitated and when you start doing things like those on the course, she calms down. I find it [the approach] often calms clients down when they are agitated.

M.E.: Do you think the training has given you other things to try?

Nurse: Yeah. Although it's a bit more difficult on nightshift because you've not got that length of time that I did before on days. You can't sit there and see what they're doing all the time.

M.E.: Can I ask you about the resident that you tried AI with? Do you think it had any impact on her daily life?

Nurse: When I was doing the training we all noticed that it was benefitting her. But now that I'm on nights, I couldn't say. I try to do it when I remember but sometimes I'm tired.

M.E.: Do you think it has had an effect on the way you view the residents overall?

Nurse: Yeah. We take communication for granted and even though some of the residents can't communicate verbally we take for granted that they understand. When you take the non-verbal approach using touch and things like that we can see that they pay more attention and the focus is on you and them. It's hard to do – everyone would have to be able to do it and learn how to do it and want to take the time out to do it for it to be workable. If they're short staffed, they might not be able to do it. ... They might not have the time.

M.E.: What other obstacles do you think there might be in passing it on to someone else?

Nurse: Well, it depends on their view. They might think what a load of nonsense or that kind of thing. Or it could be that I don't have enough time to show other members of staff. Also the problem of staffing levels. They're the kind of obstacles. All the nurses should do it. ... It seems to be helping to calm them [people with dementia] down or helping with personal care.

M.E.: What do you think would make other people take AI on board?

Nurse: Being honest – going on the course. When I first started I thought this is never going to work. And then obviously when you look back at the video and things like that, you see it working. And even families seen [sic] it working.

M.E.: Could you see it being more widely used?

Nurse: Yeah. Obviously because of the illness, people are going to deteriorate communication-wise. There is [sic] a lot of new carers, young carers that don't understand dementia. When I first started at seventeen I didn't understand, I didn't know anything about it and you just copied everybody else. Whereas we should train everyone, the new ones [unqualified staff] and the nurses [qualified] and even the older ones who are set in their ways, then things could change.

THE FUTURE OF ADAPTIVE INTERACTION

The opinions voiced by the trainee in this chapter undoubtedly shaped how we developed our training in AI. It seemed that although the overall impact of the training course was extremely positive, at the six month follow-up AI was rarely used and that the approach was not being passed on to others. This seemed odd to us because we had received such positive feedback at the time of the training from trainees, management and family members alike. Perhaps the biggest barrier to using AI in the care environment was what happened post-training; specifically, keeping AI going in care and making it part of daily life. The trainees seemed to believe that AI was an 'extra' thing that they could do, and that outside of protected training time there was no other time to engage in it. Trainees appeared to believe that AI was therefore yet another task they were being asked to do rather than viewing it as a way of being with people with advanced dementia.

The above interview suggested to us that in order for staff to maintain AI in their practice, they needed to witness more clearly the benefits for themselves as well as their clients. As a result of the above follow-up findings, our AI training includes how to include it in daily care routines. For example, we recommend that communication is assessed when a person enters a new unit, and that if a person is non-verbal this is indicated in their notes. We also advise that all nursing and care staff in a unit are trained to use AI and that each person's communication repertoire is documented. This helps the whole care team to maintain a consistent approach and also be alert to changes in a person's non-verbal communication which may warrant further investigation. To illustrate the practicalities of AI, we also explore possible care scenarios within which using the principles of AI might help to avoid distress or discomfort during routine activities, such as before, during and after personal care. Another essential element in the successful implementation of AI is the training of senior staff, including managers, who have the power to develop a structure for integrating AI into routine practice as well as providing time for training and peer support.

SUMMARY

We believe that AI has the potential to change the face of advanced dementia care by changing attitudes, improving quality of life and illuminating communicative potential. By including people with advanced dementia in the social world by using their own language we can alleviate the social isolation that these individuals experience on a daily basis. However, it is clear that in order for AI to be widely implemented, we must first regard communication in people with advanced dementia as both possible and significant. As such, we continue to research the impact of the approach and to train nursing and care staff in the principles of AI. We are hopeful that AI will contribute to a future sea change in how we view and work with individuals with advanced dementia.

REFERENCES

Caldwell, P. (2008) 'Intensive Interaction: Getting in Touch with a Child with Severe Autism.' In S. Zeedyk (ed.), *Techniques for Promoting Social Engagement in Individuals with Communicative Impairments.* London: Jessica Kingsley Publishers.

Caldwell, P. and Horwood, J. (2007) *From Isolation to Intimacy: Making Friends without Words.* London: Jessica Kingsley Publishers.

Ellis, M.P. and Astell, A.J. (2008) 'Promoting Communication with People with Severe Dementia.' In S. Zeedyk (ed.), *Techniques for Promoting Social Engagement in Individuals with Communicative Impairments.* London: Jessica Kingsley Publishers.

Ellis, M. and Astell, A. (2017a) 'Communicating with people living with dementia who are non-verbal: The creation of Adaptive Interaction.' *PloS one 12,* 8, e0180395.

Ellis, M. and Astell, A. (2017b) *Adaptive Interaction and Dementia: How to Communicate Without Speech.* London: Jessica Kingsley Publishers.

Hewett, D. (1996) 'How to do Intensive Interaction.' In M. Collis and P. Lacey (eds), *Interactive Approaches to Teaching: A Framework for INSET.* London: David Fulton Publishers.

Nind, M. (1996) 'Efficacy of Intensive Interaction: Developing sociability and communication in people with severe and complex learning difficulties using an approach based on care-giver-infant interaction.' *European Journal of Special Educational Needs 11,* 1, 48–66.

Chapter Ten
....

What We Have Communicated and What Next!

INTRODUCTION

When we first had the idea for this book there were several important considerations. First, we wanted to provide written practical guidance which was accessible to care-givers on how to speak, listen and interact with people with dementia (PWD). Although not wanting it to be too academic, we wanted to ensure this guidance was based on sound evidence, taking account of some of the recent major trials in the area which examined interventions for people engaging in behaviours that challenge (BtC), such as WHELD (Ballard *et al.*, 2018) and Challenge DEMCARE (Moniz-Cook *et al.*, 2017).

Second, we wanted to emphasise the importance of training and supervision for care-givers, these features are highlighted in the NICE guidelines (2018). Surr and colleagues's recent survey of UK training programmes clarified what successful training programmes should consist of, in terms of length and content (Surr *et al.*, 2017).

Third, we wanted to emphasise that, while working with PWD may well be complex, one can go a long way in maintaining and improving people's wellbeing via the use of good communication skills: skills that we all have knowledge of. In relation to complexity, there are times when specialist interventions are required and on these occasions the use of formulations have been found to be effective in understanding and reducing PWD's stress and distress (James and Moniz-Cook, 2018).

In specific terms, this summary chapter attempts to make the following points. These issues have been discussed in greater depth within the preceding chapters.

- All interactions permit an opportunity to provide a therapeutic intervention. Interventions, whether helping with an activity of daily living (ADL) or providing a structured therapy, are effective when they meet people's needs.

- There are a finite number of basic needs; we have identified eight in this book. When people's needs are met it enhances their wellbeing, reduces their stress and distress, and prevents the triggering of BtC.

- Connectivity is one of the main people skills for care-givers; feeling connected is crucial for everyone's wellbeing. In this book we have described several protocols designed to enhance connectiveness: customer care skills, Verbal Judo, RAM and BANGS.

- When working in people's intimate space one needs to know particularly good techniques. Helpful examples of these techniques have been provided using the PAL Instrument (Pool, 2012) and the work of Teepa Snow (Snow, 2012).

- Complex cases require more of a biopsychosocial perspective in which care-givers must utilise more background information about the nature of dementia and the person. Such cases often require a formulation to understand someone's specific needs and to find ways to meet them.

DISCUSSION

This book has highlighted that caring for PWD involves helping them maintain their independence for as long as possible, and when assistance is required we should work alongside them to meet their needs. This sometimes will involve assisting PWD with intimate care activities such as washing, use of bathroom and dressing. Input at this level can be referred to as task-oriented work, but this does not need to be the case.

For example, if the intimate care is provided in a way that enhances the PWD's wellbeing, the task can be seen as a therapeutic intervention. The role of the care-giver necessitates close and intimate contact, and we have suggested in Communication and Interaction Training (CAIT) that such contact provides the opportunity for meaningful engagement. As one of the care-givers said to us in one of our CAIT training programmes, *As a carer you've got no choice but to touch people in delicate places, so why not make such contact good and reassuring.*

In our clinical work with CAIT we have observed that some care-givers are better than others at providing positive and therapeutic interactions, and it is from these observations that we have developed the CAIT framework. Interestingly many of the good care-givers are unaware of their positive styles of engagement, therefore part of our role has been to get them to identify and articulate their skills in delivering good care. In Table 10.1 (James and Jackman, 2017), we were able to show that after attending a CAIT training programme staff became better able to articulate their skills. In the scientific literature this transformation is called moving from a state of 'unconscious competence' to one of 'conscious competence'.

Table 10.1: Articulation of skills pre- and post-CAIT Training

Staff were asked the skills they used when delivering person-centred care for people with dementia	
Prior to CAIT	**After CAIT**
Be patient	**Verbal**
Good listener	Lower your voice
Introduce yourself	Give your name so as to get trust
Good eye contact	Use simple short sentences
Collect risk information	Don't outpace
Work with the resident	Ask open questions – don't put them into a corner
Do a life story/care plans	Don't ask impossible questions
Get to know the person	Don't demand relationships if they don't recognise you
Go in twos	Use empathy/validation at times of distress
Stand the right way – eye level	Listen for cues – when in doubt say 'Tell me about it'
Don't patronise	Repeat things in different ways
Be natural	Avoid confrontations – avoid don'ts (Don't do that!)
Respect their choices	**Non-verbal**
Agree with them	Know their field of vision and stand in this visual field
Keep calm	Approach from front
Work as a team	Use more sign-language, and less speaking
Take account of poor hearing and sight	Slower pacing
Speak slowly	Slow pace, and use less words
Read the care plan	Be aware of person's public/personal space
Know their history	Approach slowly, let their brains catch up
Be at same level when talking	Use old memory tracts
Ask for help when needed	Use the sequence: visual, verbal, touch
Have knowledge of dementia	Get their attention – connect before you touch
Use their likes to get them to do things	Give them time to focus and recognise
	Body language needs to be non-confronting
	Develop incompatible behaviours – the person cannot be holding their penis if you've asked him to hold a bath sponge for you
	Be aware of hypersensitivity, hand on shoulder
	Use the Hand-under-Hand™ technique (Snow, 2012)
	General
	Use your knowledge of the type of dementia
	Use knowledge of their strengths and weaknesses
	Distract them if stuck in a particular time frame
	Don't overload their brain
	Distract and redirect
	Take account of person's timeline (how old does he think he is?)
	Avoid accidental cueing – saying goodbye at end of shift, putting on your coat

Our analysis of good care has shown that it usually occurs when the care-givers are meeting PWD's basic needs. We have identified these needs as: physical comfort and freedom from pain; perception of safety; positive touch; love and belonging; esteem needs; control over environment and possessions; fun; occupation and exploration.

We believe that positive interventions routinely satisfy one or more of these needs, and highly effective interventions satisfy many of the needs simultaneously. Although our identification of needs has not been validated empirically, it is interesting to see how closely they match with similar models of wellbeing (see Fox *et al.*, 2005 and MAREP, Power, 2014). Fox and Powers' wellbeing frameworks are illustrated in Table 10.2.

Table 10.2: Frameworks of basic needs

Fox *et al.* (2005) Domains of wellbeing	MAREP (Power, 2014) meaningful leisure experiences	James and Jackman (2017) basic needs
Identity	Being me	Esteem needs
Connectedness	Being with	Love and belonging
		Positive touch
Autonomy	Seeking freedom	Control over environment and possessions
Security	Finding balance	Perception of safety
Meaning	Making a difference	Occupation and
Growth	Growing and developing	exploration
Joy	Having fun	Fun
		Physical comfort and freedom from pain

One feature of our model that is different from many other frameworks is that it highlights that in dementia care the needs are not so egocentric. In fact, the stress experienced by many PWD is because of their worries about the safety and wellbeing of other people (*Is my wife okay?; I have to get back home to cook their dinner; My child will be waiting for me*). It is often the stress associated with concerns about other people's needs that leads to the distress.

As we, and others, have argued when people have their basic needs met it enhances their wellbeing, reduces their stress and distress, and prevents the triggering of BtC (Algase *et al.*, 1996; Power, 2014; Scottish Government, 2017). This conceptualisation is well understood, and we frequently see services or care providers describing their interventions as being needs-led. However, our experience is that when you ask employees of such services what they mean by the term needs-led, the employees provide vague responses. Such vagueness often results in a lack of clear goals in relation to actions and treatments within care teams.

It was for this reason we wanted to identify a specific list of needs, which could then act as a checklist in care settings to see whether there were actions and interventions care-planned to meet each need. Further, it allowed us to treat people engaging in BtC when we had very little background information about them. In such circumstances we could simply go down our checklist, ensuring there were specific actions aligned to meet each need (James and Jackman, 2017).

The importance of having meaningful connections is topical and draws our attention to the fascinating field of social neuroscience (Cacioppo, Berntson and Decety, 2010). The essence of this field is the hypothesis that the human brain has evolved as a social organ. In other words, a lot of the newer parts of the brain (frontal lobes) have developed to promote effective communication and interaction (coordination of speech, comprehension, problem-solving, insight, theory of mind and empathy). Further, the scientists in this field think that we should not assess the functioning of a person's brain in isolation, rather examine its performance in a social situation to determine its true capabilities.

A key hypothesis is that when a brain is starved of stimulation and human interaction it will not function well, and further skills will be lost if the mind remains isolated for a prolonged period. This issue is crucial in the case of dementia, particularly if care-givers do not attempt to communicate with PWD regularly. In such cases the organic deficits may worsen because of an overlay of functional difficulties.

In some of the early chapters of this book we examined several protocols developed to enhance connectiveness and people's senses of control and dignity. We borrowed from the customer care skills of the high street and the Verbal Judo techniques of the North American police (Thompson and Jenkins, 2013). Thompson's work is particularly inspiring as it describes his journey from being a potential bully to an expert communicator in the practical role of being a police officer in the USA. He recognised that it was vital for a police officer to know how to negotiate and deal with violence under pressure in a professional manner. Borrowing from such work, we would like our care-givers to know what interactions are helpful, check they have been helpful and be able to adjust their approaches accordingly.

On reflection, we are surprised that very few health settings have adopted such programmes; one could surely argue that keeping PWD happy is just as important as maintaining the wellbeing of shoppers. We also illustrated Macaulay's BANGS approach and RAM, both of which have proven extremely popular in our CAIT teaching sessions. The techniques appear to provide memorable steps, giving the care-givers a sense of confidence and control in situations that they previously found difficult to manage.

While the protocols are useful guides in situations where a care-giver does not necessarily know the PWD well, tailored interactions and interventions are often more effective. When care-givers tailor approaches based on someone's history and specific needs, this is often referred to as providing person-centred care. Person-centred practices are frequently structured around biopsychosocial frameworks, in which a knowledge of the type of dementia, physical issues (biological aspects), the person's premorbid personality, likes and dislikes (psychological aspects), and the impact of the environment on the person (social aspects) are all considered.

In this book we have been realistic and practical, stating clearly that in complex presentations, including when PWD's behaviours are severe or risky, medication may be required (also see James and Jackman, 2017; NICE, 2018). Current guidance requires care-givers to consider, however, using some form of non-pharmacological intervention before resorting to drugs. Unfortunately, the evidence base for many of these non-pharmacological interventions is rather poor, and the findings from the studies inconsistent (see Ballard *et al.*, 2018; NICE, 2018).

To make sense of these inconsistencies within the CAIT framework we have suggested that in the past there has often been a misunderstanding of the goals of many of our psychological approaches (i.e. we became fixated on the type of approach rather than the function of what it was trying to achieve). As we explained in Chapter 6, we believe that a goal of an intervention should not be to deliver a set therapy such as music, aromatherapy, doll or animal assisted, rather to target our eight basic needs. In other words, we believe the therapies are vehicles for meeting needs, and should therefore be designed better as a way of doing this.

RESEARCH

The WHELD programme (Ballard *et al.*, 2018; Fossey *et al.* 2014) demonstrated that treating PWD as individuals, talking to them about their interests and their lives, and tailoring activities to things they enjoy had a small but important positive effect on their lives and additionally showed some reduction in BtC. As part of this project the researchers undertook a major review of BtC interventions to determine which they would use in their experimental phase of their study. We believe it was telling that the researchers failed to find consistent enough evidence for a particular type of therapy, and so in their final experimental phase employed rather generic interventions, such as person-centred care and social interaction.

With highly complex cases, PWD's needs may be difficult to identify and in such situations we have described how to undertake a formulation, which attempts to understand and meet someone's specific needs. Formulations are recommended as the gold-standard approach for the treatment of BtC (James and Moniz-Cook, 2018), but do require training and supervision in the support of their use.

The Challenge DEMCARE programme examined whether such teaching could be undertaken using an online-training methodology (Moniz-Cook *et al.*, 2017). It examined the management of BtC at home and in care homes. Its care home intervention (Challenge ResCare) targeted PWD and clinically significant BtC, meaning that this intervention focused on more severe cases of dementia-related behavioural symptoms. Care home 'Staff Champions' received training facilitated by a dementia nurse trainer using an e-learning interactive course and real-life films of cases of BtC and behavioural expressions of distress to learn the detective skills needed for individually tailored health and psychosocial interventions for PWD.

The dementia nurse trainer then worked with staff to develop case-specific health and psychosocial interventions for those with clinically significant challenging behaviour. Following training, levels of challenging behaviour in people with clinically significant BtC reduced, but this effect did not last (Moniz-Cook *et al.*, 2017). A review of the findings led the researchers to emphasise the importance of the interpersonal element in training of BtC skills, which in some ways may mirror the connectiveness we have discussed earlier in terms of relationships with PWD.

The findings of DEMCARE, and WHELD, strengthen the case for individually formulated interventions, often involving detective work and testing different ways of interacting with the PWD. They also confirm that, to deliver effective complex interventions for BtC, ongoing support from an external therapist is often required. This is particularly relevant for those with clinically significant BtC where fluctuations in behaviour may occur due to changes in a person's health and environmental circumstances.

RECOMMENDATIONS

In an earlier book the first author (James, 2011) stated that caring for PWD is highly complex work, perhaps some of the most complex work one could ever undertake in terms of health and social care delivery.

For example, in addition to dealing with people's emotional difficulties, mental health issues and physical frailty, one must also do this with people with major declining cognitive skills, who may be residing in environments either they do not recognise or where they do not want to be. Owing to the complexity, James was keen to acknowledge the skills inherent in many caregiving practices. He suggested structuring the approaches and labelling them as therapies; he even outlined the contents of a potential course.

Hence, our major recommendation from this book returns to the above theme. We suggest that from the material outlined in this textbook an accredited teaching course is developed. The contents of the course will need to be broadened, incorporating material from other programmes such as the Dementia Training Standards Framework (Health Education England, 2018) or VIPS (Brooker, 2007) to achieve a standardised curriculum. Ideally the course should be endorsed by a national or professional body. This would ensure credibility and wide dissemination, and it could form the backbone of professionals' induction programmes.

The second recommendation, to further endorse CAIT's credibility and value, must be a vigorous assessment of its impact. Helpful models for such evaluation have been provided by the empirical assessments of Dementia Care Mapping (van de Ven *et al.*, 2014) and VIPS (Brooker, 2007).

CONCLUSION

There are numerous manuals on how to support care-givers who are working with PWD (Brooker, 2007; Sheard, 2008; Teri, 2009; Fossey *et al.*, 2017) which stress the importance of effective interpersonal interactions. As with this book, these manuals are attempting to move carers from states of unconscious competence (or incompetence) to one of conscious competence in terms of their roles as carers. In the latter state, the care-givers will gain self-awareness of the relevant attitudes, knowledge and skills required to be able to communicate across a range of situations.

In the early part of this book we learned the importance of having a thoughtful and structured approach to communicating. Indeed, appreciating that we often need to consciously change the way we communicate is an important first step. This is clearly not a novel scenario because we are constantly altering our communication styles, for example, when interacting with young children, high status or low status individuals or drunks! What may be novel, however, is thinking clearly about what constitutes good, clear and respectful communication. To aid us in doing this we have borrowed from training programmes used both in industry and public services.

Next we provided information about dementia and the sensory deficits related to cognitive impairment in order to help care-givers understand and empathise with the experiences of PWD. We were keen to show that PWD are often interpreting information differently during their attempts to navigate their way round their environments, and they will be using degraded information owing to their problem-solving deficits as they attempt to steer their course. As we say in our teaching *'It important for us to recognise that PWD are more restricted in the information available to them when working out what's going on.'* When discussing empathy, we were clear that simply empathising with people's distress could be unhelpful, perhaps even demotivating, if it does not guide us to actions that meet PWD's needs.

Later we described the CAIT's hub in more detail and showed that different approaches were needed by care-givers to assist them to structure their responses, using protocols and simple techniques. In the final section on CAIT we recommended that specialist support was needed to assist in challenging situations, and we provided examples of the use of a formulation-led approach (Newcastle Framework).

Notwithstanding the nature of the job or role, whether one is using complex formulations or protocols or supporting someone in the bathroom, the core of the activity is meeting people's needs and achieving this via effective communication and interaction. Indeed, we should treat each contact with the PWD as a way of connecting positively. The person may not always remember what has been exchanged between the two of you, but the sense of overall wellbeing will be carried over and their good mood will become more pervasive.

In Chapters 7, 8 and 9, experts in their respective fields introduced us to new perspectives in communication. Thwaites described the work of Teepa Snow who has revolutionised the area with her practical approach to communication. Thwaites gave us case studies of situations which required care-givers to provide intimate care, and the methods being described demonstrated a degree of overlap between Snow's Positive Approach to Care™ (PAC™) approach and CAIT. This chapter is particularly welcome because most of Snow's training to date has been by workshops and DVDs, and very little written material is available. Tanner's contribution, Chapter 8, draws our attention to the nature and role of touch in dementia care. This chapter is partially a summary of his book and highlights this fundamental aspect of care, and how to ensure it can be done effectively and positively. In the penultimate chapter, Ellis and Astell provided us with information in the much neglected area of communicating with people in the very late stages of dementia. They have fused practical approaches and research to enhance their methods.

Finally, much of the work, perhaps all, outlined in this book is nicely summarised in a quote we came across in a promotional leaflet by a national UK department store by Emma Marchant (2017): 'Engaging with people who live with dementia is largely about communication…and how you make them feel emotionally.' This is a key theme of the store in developing a dementia-friendly workforce. This again highlights that the care sector can learn much from other organisations in their approaches to communication and interactions, perhaps even in the area of dementia.

REFERENCES

Algase, D.L., Beck, C., Kolanowski, A., Whall, A. *et al.* (1996) 'Need-driven dementia compromised behavior: An alternative view of disruptive behavior.' *American Journal of Alzheimer's Disease 11*, 10, 12–19.

Ballard, C., Corbett, A., Orrell, M. *et al.* (2018) 'Impact of person-centred care training and person-centred activities on quality of life, agitation, and antipsychotic use in people with dementia living in nursing homes: A cluster-randomised controlled trial.' *PLoS Med 15*, 2, e1002500.

Brooker, D. (2007) *Person-Centred Dementia Care: Making Services Better.* London: Jessica Kingsley Publishers.

Cacioppo, J.T., Berntson, G. and Decety, J. (2010) 'Social neuroscience and its relationship to social psychology.' *Social Cognition 28*, 6, 675–685.

Fossey, J., Masson, S., Stafford, J., Lawrence, V., Corbett, A. and Ballard, C. (2014) 'The disconnect between evidence and practice: A systematic review of person-centred interventions and training manuals for care home staff working with people with dementia.' *International Journal of Geriatric Psychiatry 29*, 797–807.

Fox, N., Norton, L., Rashap, A. *et al.* (2005) 'Wellbeing: Beyond quality of life.' Now available as 'The Eden Alternative Domains of Wellbeing: Revolutionizing the experience of home by bringing wellbeing to life.' Available at www.edenalt.org, accessed on October 06, 2018.

Health Education England (2018) Dementia Training Standard Framework. Available at www.hee.nhs.uk/our-work/dementia-awareness/core-skills, accessed on October 05, 2018.

James, I.A. (2011) *Understanding Behaviour in Dementia that Challenges.* London: Jessica Kingsley Publishers.

James, I.A. and Jackman, L. (2017) *Understanding Behaviour in Dementia that Challenges.* 2nd edn. London: Jessica Kingsley Publishers.

James, I.A. and Moniz-Cook, E. (2018) 'Behaviours that challenge in dementia: A briefing paper for British Psychological Society.' Available at www.bps.org.uk/sites/bps.org.uk/files/Policy%20-%20Files/Evidence%20briefing%20-%20behaviour%20that%20challenges%20in%20dementia.pdf, accessed on October 06, 2018.

Marchant, E. (2017) 'The Partner Driving Dementia Awareness at John Lewis.' Available at www.johnlewis.com/my-john-lewis-insider-news/dementia-story, accessed on September 18, 2018.

Moniz-Cook, E., Hart, C., Woods, B., Whitaker, C. *et al.* (2017) 'Challenge Demcare: Management of challenging behaviour in dementia at home and in care homes: Development, evaluation and implementation of an online individualised intervention for care homes; and a cohort study of specialist community mental health care for families.' *Programme Grants for Applied Research 5*, 15. Available at www.ncbi.nlm.nih.gov/pubmed/28783270, accessed on September 18, 2018.

NICE (2018) 'Dementia: Assessment, management and support for people living with dementia and their carers' Guidance/ng 97.

Pool, J. (2012) *The Pool Activity Level (PAL) Instrument for Occupational Profiling: A Practical Resource for Carers of People with Cognitive Impairment (Bradford Dementia Group Good Practice Guides).* 4th edn. London: Jessica Kingsley Publishers.

Power, A. (2014) *Dementia Beyond Disease: Enhancing Wellbeing.* Baltimore, MD: Health Profession Press.

Scottish Government (2017) Scotland's National Dementia Strategy 2017–2020. The Scottish Government. Available at www.alzscot.org/assets/0002/6035/Third_Dementia_Strategy.pdf, accessed on October 06, 2018.

Sheard, D. (2008) 'Growing: training that works in dementia care.' Alzheimer Society, UK.

Snow, T. (2012) *Dementia Care-Giver Guide: Teepa Snow's Positive Approach Techniques for Care-giving, Alzheimer's and Other Forms of Dementia.* Mason, OH: Cedar Village.

Surr, C., Gates, C., Irving, D. *et al.* (2017) 'Effective dementia education and training for the health and social care workforce: A systematic review of the literature.' *Review Education Research 87*, 5, 966–1002.

Teri, L., Huda, P., Gibbons, L., Young, H. and van Leynseele, J. (2005) 'STAR: A dementia-specific training program for staff in assisted living residences.' *The Gerontologist 45*, 5, 686–693.

Thompson, G. and Jenkins. J. (2013) *Verbal Judo: The Gentle Art of Persuasion.* New York: HarperCollins Press.

van de Ven, G., Draskovic, I., van Herpen, E., Koopmans, R.T., Donders, R., Zuidema, S.U. Vernooij-Dassen, M.J. (2014) 'The economics of dementia-care mapping in nursing homes: A cluster-randomised controlled trial.' *PloS One 9*, 1, e86662.

Subject Index

Author Index